ONE *SPLIT* SECOND

SUZAN BRYAN HOPPE, AAI, AAM, CPIW

Robbie Dean Press
Ann Arbor

Printed in the U.S.A.

ISBN: 0-9630608-3-X

PROLOGUE

One split second is all it takes to blink your eye, to snap your finger. Nine-year-old Danny Hoppe ran across a busy road June 10, 1982. He was struck by a van going 45 miles per hour. The second his head hit the hood, the resulting Traumatic Brain Injury, "TBI" changed Danny's and the family's life, forever.

September 20, 1990, 47-year-old Suzan Hoppe, Danny's Mom, suffered an interventricular, intercerebral aneurysm in the right frontal lobe. Another second, another change, but still the family goes on, grateful for every new opportunity afforded by future seconds, now more valuable and prized, in light of what could have been.

My message is that although your life is altered, it can still go on. You may have to change your dream and your perspective. You adjust, adapt and you look for new avenues to meet the new goals. Focus changes. Hope is like a lighthouse. It is like a beacon. We keep trying to stay in its light. Although doctors will tell you not to have false hope; however, hope and faith is all we have and we MUST hold on. It gets you through that bad time.

The head-injured person dies and a new person emerges. The change can be dramatic. You say goodbye to the person that was and learn to love the person that is now.

The statistics of head injury are staggering: 700,000 each year in the United States--100,000 die and 70,000 to 90,000 people are permanently disabled as the result.

Serious head injuries usually result in prolonged loss of consciousness or coma. While some are brief, others last days or weeks. The longer the coma, the more difficulties may occur which require rehabilitation for speech impairment, intellectual deficits, behavioral disorder, and physical disabilities. The rehab period may go on for years, and some may be impaired to such a degree it may be a long time, or they may never return to a regular life.

Spontaneous Intracranial Hemorrhages strike most frequently the 35- to 55-year-old. Cerebrovascular accidents (CVA's) account for approximately 20% of all strokes. Intracerebral hemorrhage (ICH) commonly afflicts older adults with a history of hypertension. But patients as young of 20 or 30 with arteriovenous malformations (AVM) also suffer such hemorrhages.

The U. S. Department of Health and Human Services estimate there are 500,000 of these annually. Many of these also require long-term therapy for cognitive and physical impairment.

When we combine the two populations, one million people annually will suffer some type of insult to the brain. If the average family is 2.5 people, then two-and-a-half million people each year will be impacted by this trauma.

Why should you read this book? To know you are not alone. Maybe it will hold the promise of hope and dispel the fear that life will never be good again; or that you will never laugh, the only display of emotion will be tears of anger or heart-wrenching pain.

It could even banish from your vocabulary the term "False Hope". In my opinion, that is an Oxymoran. Hope is eternal and it is not true or false. It is just what it says, "Hope". We all need it to survive, to attain, to not only overcome, but conquer adversity. It is never, never false.

There are never two traumatic brain injuries the same. The only thing that is homogeneous about this "Silent Epidemic" is the havoc it wrecks on the family. But that too, with love, nuturing, compassion, fresh insight, a lot of courage and a dash of humor, can bring you out of the darkness which is this injury and into the light which is tomorrow.

DEDICATION

There is not a night, nor a place, darker or more fearsome than a confused mind. I would like to dedicate this book to the following people who have, in their own special ways, been "a Point of Light" in that dark place: Jeanne Axelrod, AKA Nana, to those who love this tiny, but mighty, Jewish lady. She, not only through her fierce protection of those she cares about, brings light and love, but she also gave the world Marilyn Hope Axelrod, now Koster, who, through her continued belief in miracles as a Speech Pathologist, gave my son, Danny, back to the world. Through her skills and friendship, she continues to work toward giving the world back to me.

Since this is my book, I assume the dedication may go on. There was another lady who brought light into my life when, as a troubled teenager, I was not sure life was worth it. Her love and understanding carried me through those very dark years. Many years older, hair now white, with steps a little slower, but arms still long enough to encircle every needy child within her hearing, my aunt, Dora Bryan.

And to my son, Danny, whose story this really is. Without you, I might not be able to write about either of us. You truly have been and continue to be, "The Wind Beneath My Wings".

> My religion consists of a humble admiration of the illimitable superior spirit who reveals himself in the slight details we are able to perceive with our frail and feeble minds.
>
> --Einstein

CHAPTER 1

Mother's Day, 1991. We returned to a sitting position in the pew after singing the Doxology. Our Pastor was reading Scripture, and I was gazing at the cross, lost in my own conversation with God, which I do occasionally during the service (this, I hope pleases my Pastor when he reads it). The dark wood of the cross often draws me; and, as I sat there between two of my sons, David, 25 and Danny, 18, I reflected on how at times earlier in their lives I had released them from my loving, but not always capable care, and laid them in the arms of God--whose care is always perfect--for him to make the choice: to take them back, as they were only on loan to me anyway, or heal them and let me have them in my life awhile longer.

I thought about David, who had suffered brain damage at birth from lack of oxygen which was not discovered until, at nine months, he began having Grand

Mal seizures. I would hold his tiny, writhing body and pray for him to get through it. At age two, by then to all appearances a healthy baby, he suddenly went from one seizure to another. Because I was home alone, I called the Michigan State Police; and very shortly, a trooper screeched into my driveway to take us to the hospital. He was a very young officer, and I'm sure the drive was much more taxing on him than me because of my many months' past experience with the seizures. His furtive glances and statements of, "Ma'am, is the baby okay?", were not appreciated by this mother until years later. All I could say was, "Get this car going faster", and, "Just get us to the hospital".

That he did, and David's neurologist, Dr. Alan Clague, met me at the Emergency entrance, took the baby from my arms and told me to "find a seat", he'd be with me as soon as there was something he could tell me.

I collapsed in a chair, the adrenaline that had kept me going subsided and left room for the fear, tears and shaking, which took over my body. My little boy was in a room with virtual strangers. What if he got scared? What if there were more seizures? What if, my God, he died?

A not-often-thought-about advantage of youth is that death doesn't impact us at age twenty as it does when we get older and more appreciative of life. I knew I could lose him, but there was not the terror that I would learn about sixteen years later.

David had pneumonia, the series of seizures was caused by a 106-degree temperature and they were going to admit him. It was hard for me to reconcile pneumonia, which I had always perceived as very serious with the person acting sick, with this two-year-old child who, that very morning, had emptied a whole box of Oxydol on the kitchen floor to run his cars through. Hyperactivity was also a problem we had to deal with, but it was so hard to believe this little boy, so apparently healthy and getting into mischief two hours earlier, was headed for an oxygen tent.

St. Joseph Mercy Hospital, run by The Sisters of Mercy in 1965, was a combination of aging structure and additions. As I walked through the halls and saw the faith symbols and the changing architecture, I remember thinking of the comparison between new and old, and how the old was slowly giving way to the new in much the same way as people we often try in our human-ness to release the old to make way for the new, knowing we will someday pass from sight--like the old hospital building.

I reached David's room and sat in a chair next to the bed and, as I searched the face of my sleeping son, asked God not to take him. If it had to be someone, let it be me. I had lived for 21 years while he had not had an opportunity to have any life. "Please God, take me."

David rallied. He was soon crawling out of the crib--so often in fact, they had put him into a gown that tied to the bed. The nurses, although they liked his hugs, were not happy as his energy returned.

One night, after seeing he was asleep, I left the room and standing before a very large crucifix, I let go of David. Even though he was now well, the reality of the past two weeks had begun to sink in. Children with seizures that are uncontrolled get progressively worse. More damage is done to the brain with each severe series. But my heart knew that other children would ostracize my son. Even worse than the tormenting and name calling, the teasing of young school children might, in fact, be even more hurtful than just being left alone. With these thoughts tumbling around in my head, along with the fear of losing my job and having no medical coverage to pay the hospital bills which were mounting, I fell to my knees and gave David willingly over into God's care. If, in fact, he would not outgrow the seizures as expected, if he would be pained by cutting remarks, then I would gladly give him up. As soon as I said those things a feeling of peace came over me. What a valuable lesson I learned, a lesson that would guide me through many more years to come.

Back in the pew at church, Danny, sitting on the other side of me, reached over and took my hand. The tears welled in my eyes as I remembered the morning I had laid him as well in God's loving arms.

When we sat through the long first night as Danny struggled for life but was no better, I stood at the window in the hospital's Intensive Care waiting room watching the sun rise and released him willingly to God from my care. Hours of feeling the pain that only a mother, whose own body breathed life into a child for nine months, can know the helplessness--when your body, your skills, your knowledge can do nothing for your child except watch a machine breathe life into a body that, now injured, houses the miracle that was your son.

Sitting between my sons in church, the tears freely rolled down my cheeks as I could not let go of the overwhelming emotion of sheer joy they were there--on either side of me--these two sons I could have lost but didn't, and my own life which could have ended seven months earlier, but hadn't. We had all been spared, and what a joyous Mother's Day God had given me.

The great philosopher Plato has noted that as we climb toward the apex of the triangle of our lives, as the base gets smaller and smaller, at the pinnacle, at the very top, there is only room for one primary commitment.

If it is not apparent by now, my pinnacle is and has been for some time, my faith. I wouldn't now, nor have I ever tried to impose that on other people, but it is the thread, interwoven in my life, that has kept the fabric strong. Whatever yours, may it strengthen you, and may you have extra to share with that person who needs you now more than ever, to keep hope alive within yourself and him/her.

In the darkest hour the soul is replenished and given strength to continue and endure.

--Heart Warrior Chosa

CHAPTER 2

It was a warm, sunny June day. School would be over tomorrow, and I'm sure Danny was not the only fourth-grader who was anticipating that freedom you never again felt as much as that which is enjoyed as a child the last day of school.

Doug and I were in the office, caught between our current staff person moving away because of her husband's job offer and a new one expected the coming Monday.

The phone rang. It was our son David. Out of breath, near tears, he said, "Mom, Danny's been hit on Saline-Ann Arbor Road. Police are there. You need to come."

Danny, Doug's and my only child. (Doug had three children and I had two when we married ten years before.) Danny, the child I had convinced him to have through salesmanship, pleading and, finally, tears, was hurt. How badly I did not know and did not want to think about. I had to get there. I hollered at Doug who was in his office, to get the car keys--we had to leave--and I apologized to the customer who had been sitting across from me when the call came in. "We're closing right now. Our son has been hit by a car." I hoped she understood.

We left the office and I was torn between wanting to hurry and what was safe. Those six miles became the longest in my life, and traffic was backed up because of the police cars and ambulance which kept us too far away.

Doug got out from behind the wheel and ran towards where Danny lay. I slid over into the driver's seat and drove on the shoulder until I could see the people huddled over Danny's body. I shut the car off and, as I approached, a big policeman blocked my path. I couldn't go see my son. He wouldn't let me over there. Anger mounted as I prepared to go through or over him to get to Danny. But before I could put my thoughts into action, they were putting Danny on a stretcher and walking toward the ambulance. Doug indicated he was riding with Danny, and I ran back to our car, determined to follow. And follow I did. As close as I dared, stopping only long enough for red lights in downtown Ann Arbor, to insure it was clear before proceeding. Every light was red, and I ran them all. Once again, adrenaline was keeping me going. There were no tears, just sheer determination that I WOULD be with my son at the hospital and, in my ignorance of the injury to his nine-year-old body, KNEW he'd be just fine.

I lost the ambulance in campus traffic and then made a wrong turn, so by the time I slid into a parking space at the Emergency entrance, the triage team had met the ambulance at the door and whisked my baby away. I was not to see him for eight more hours.

But while Doug and I sat in a room behind a closed door where family could gather and with a telephone so we could make and receive calls, over the next eight hours Danny's plight would be made as clear to us as our minds could then accept.

Doug's manager, Harry Ahrens and his wife, Janice, were the first ones there and helped me make calls to our other children, as well as make arrangements for our oldest daughter, DeLyn, to go to the house to be with David. In my mother's heart, I knew David needed comforting, but Danny needed me more.

As I write this, an Erma Bombeck column I once read spoke about "Mom's Favorite Child" and that one was always the one who needed her most, right then. As David once needed me at the hospital, now I felt Danny needed me to be with him, even with all my ignorance.

Doug was wringing his hands and crying, the sounds of Danny moaning in the ambulance still in his ears. This child he hadn't wanted in the beginning had won him over from the day the nurse in the delivery room placed this wide-eyed, wondering baby boy in his arms.

Danny has genetically been his father's clone. The resemblance to actions, attitudes, likes and dislikes were apparent way before he was old enough to have heard stories about his father as a boy. Some other things he did were also a little unnerving: At three he told stories about his grandpa Hoppe who had passed away years before he was born--stories that only could be verified by Doug's mother. When she concurred, we certainly had something to think about for the rest of the day.

Given the fact that twice in the past Doug had suffered chest pains, now at age 54, I was afraid he'd have a heart attack if he couldn't ease the pain of Danny's trauma. I requested a sedative for him which he, for the first time in our marriage, accepted willingly. Maybe he was hoping to dull the pain he was feeling. Or maybe even hoped it would knock him out so he could descend into a blackness that would shut out everything.

For many years we've known people handle things differently. Old from young, educated, uneducated, men from women, and I had previously toyed with the idea of writing an "Injury His, Injury Hers"-type book which would validate to readers those differences are, in fact, real. We can't be another person. We can't get inside his thoughts, nor feel his pain. We only have our own feelings as reference and how often that inflicts even more pain on those we love. And for husband and wife, that spouse we vowed to be with and support through good and bad, we find ourselves withdrawing, as though by not expressing our pain it will make theirs easier to bear. I don't believe it works that way. If left to continue, a void is created that only a master bridge builder can hope to overcome.

I became the one in charge. Not so much because I was the one in our family who did that, but it became, as I look back, an instinctive survival technique. If I were running the show, it had to turn out okay. I wish I were as certain now as I had been on that June day in 1982.

The doctors and technicians were in and out of the family waiting room. I signed all the papers for all the tests as routinely as I had signed insurance applications the past ten years. They needed to do an angiogram to determine if the impact to his chest wall, which had bruised and collapsed the right lung and had then forced so much air into the left it blew out, had also damaged his heart. Cat scans were run because he was not responding, and the saucer-shaped bruise on the right side of the back of his head where it struck the hood of the van indicated a head injury. The femur in his right leg which had been broken by the bumper needed to be pinned for traction. They "really were sorry", but they "couldn't tell us much more". The surgeons were all checking him over. They were doing the best they could. Danny had been put on a respirator to keep his body alive and life-giving oxygen was supplied to the brain.

The word was spreading around Saline and Ann Arbor that Doug Hoppe's son had been hit, or Danny Hoppe had been hit, and calls started coming in. There was plenty of help fielding the calls those first hours, so I didn't have to keep repeating the same facts over and over, burning them into my brain and my heart so deeply I wasn't sure I could stand the pain.

My one resource learned in childhood was "back away". Fake it. Pretend you don't want something, keep saying you don't care 'til you don't. Act like it doesn't hurt and they'll leave you alone. These coping mechanisms, once again brought to the surface by the pain of helplessness kicked in and I moved forward. Not in a fog that covered awareness, but in a Saran-wrap existence that allowed me to see, hear, talk, take charge but not allow any more pain into my psyche. Doug's pain and anguish were visible, but mine was tucked away in a closet of my mind to be kept there until I wanted, by my own choosing, to look at it.

Danny was ready to be moved from Emergency to the Children's Intensive Care Unit. We left the safe haven of our little family waiting room to wind the hallways of University Hospital, where the Emergency room was located, to Mott Children's Hospital building where Danny would be placed in the care of some very special nurses.

No books, television show or life event had prepared me for what I saw when they finally let us in the Intensive Care Unit. Just past the baby units which were glassed in and in the first bed on the left, the first big hospital bed, lay my tiny son, all four-feet, 75 pounds of him. An IPC monitor (Intercranial Pressure Monitor) was sticking out of his head. (A hole had been drilled through his skull and an IPC monitor had been inserted to monitor pressure on the brain caused from swelling, more often than not the culprit than the original blow in a closed-head injury.) He was attached also to a monitor that kept track of heart rate and blood pressure. Two tubes protruded from under his ribs, tubes that drained fluid from around the lungs and helped keep them inflated. The respirator still pumped air into the lungs and the sound of the accordion-like part which expanded and contracted at regular intervals although artificial, was a sound of life. The right leg, suspended by a pin through the bone just above the knee, swung from the traction bar, and IV's were also supplying life-giving nourishment as well as medication to this tiny body in the big hospital bed.

They had given Danny a drug to put him, or keep him, in a coma-like state until his body could start the miracle we all take for granted--healing itself. Intelligence, what we learn, taught us long ago about bleeding--how the body starts sending out its own resources to fight infection, causes clotting, starts renewing tissue and mending broken bones. We take much of that for granted, even for something so small as a cut on our finger. What we don't think about, unless we have studied, from education, or frame-of-reference, or experienced head-injury up close, is that brain cells don't heal. They can't replicate themselves, although when brain cells are injured and die, many times other cells easily pick up their function. In some cases only time, sometimes years, is needed to restore function.

But, speaking from both sides of that scenario, not knowing is better. Think of all the things man has accomplished because he never thought he couldn't do it despite adversity and handicaps. Look who we have as examples: Helen Keller, Theodore Roosevelt, Albert Einstein and many like them who never thought they couldn't do it. Where would we be if Edison had not pursued his quest for electricity; Bell, the telephone?

Not knowing some things gave me hope. Reading books on the brain while sitting those long, awful hours in the waiting room gave me a familiarity with different areas of the brain and their function. Not quite enough to hang out a shingle and perform brain surgery, but at least I could ask questions and try to understand the answers without a look of complete bewilderment on my face.

After seeing Danny for the first time that evening, I just knew he'd sleep through the night and wake in the morning, wondering how long he'd have to stay in that bed and how long before he could play his beloved baseball again. As family and friends came and went all through the night, I talked as if it were all going to be okay. By morning, the horror would be over.

As soon as we felt it was reasonable, we went in the room. Danny would be talking to me, I knew it. But he wasn't moving. He was as unresponsive externally as he had been the night before. I left the unit, crushed inside. Outside I maintained the appearance that things would still be okay. There were calls to be made--the insurance company, a trip to be canceled, arrangements for the office, the house, Doug's mom had just had cataract surgery and she needed someone to stay with her. I found a new way to not deal with the reality that was glaring at me. If I stayed really busy, I wouldn't have to think about Danny, still asleep. That action set in motion less than 24 hours ago would stay with me for years. Keep running, and run so fast the pain can't catch you. Smart thing to do? Using the 20-20 vision we all have in hindsight, it was neither good nor bad, but I do believe it played a part in changes in my life eight years later.

Our family took over one whole side of the Intensive Care waiting room. Two daughters, Denise and Callie, slept there on chairs or the floor with us. I had no intention of leaving the hospital proper until Danny could talk to me.

Doug helped field the phone calls and cards and letters began pouring in. Danny's friends made a tape recording that we played for him. People responded to us in a way I would not have imagined. Because Doug had been born and raised in Ann Arbor and his business as an insurance agent gave him constant visibility in the paper, we received a lot of caring attention.

As I remember all of that, how blessed I feel, and realize how truly horrible it must be for those who have no one but each other as parents to a sick child. Inner strength needs nourishment, and, as human beings, it is very hard to keep going when there are only two of you who must take turns bolstering the emotional foundation of the other, to shore up the belief system that begins to waiver in the face of day-to-day sameness.

Father's Day that year was spent with our children visiting Dad in the waiting room, and all of us wanting to give him what he wanted most--Danny to wake up. It was many years later when I ran across the "Greatest Father of the Year Award", which Danny had already purchased for his Dad for that now remembered Father's Day, that I finally gave it to Doug. I couldn't bear to see his reaction to it on that Father's Day in 1982.

By that time, the neurosurgeons had told us there was severe brain-stem damage, that the impact to the head had caused the brain to move within the skull and resulted in a shearing effect. Danny was in the black, never-never-land of coma, and the prognosis was that he would never awaken.

My reading began to then focus intently on the brain stem. Who were those neurosurgeons to tell me? I watched the monitors; Doug watched the monitors. We could get no outer response, but when I talked to Danny and rubbed or patted a bare spot not covered by or stuck by something, the blood-pressure and intracranial pressure went up. When Doug talked to him, it came back down. He was responding! Because all the numbers were better for Danny at the lower level, I didn't talk much. Doug, who had been his coach in Little League as he hit home runs and snagged ground balls and finally became a pitcher, became the voice that soothed him. Doug would sit by his bed and say, "Just stay calm, pal", and relate to baseball, and Danny's body would relax and no longer swing from the traction bar. Callie would go in and read him stories during the night. I felt even more helpless, so I sat in the waiting room or stretched out on the floor at night.

When all was quiet at night, I would lay there and concentrate really hard, trying to connect on a different level with Danny. Although he was never the pal to me he was to his Dad, I thought we had had a great relationship. I would picture him in my mind on a ball field; and I knew in my heart if I could see him in my mind running again, he'd be okay.

It didn't happen--not for many nights but one night, I could see him rounding first, although it was through a green haze--as if I were looking through water. I'm sure if someone had had me hooked up to monitors at that point, my heart-rate or blood pressure would have alarmed them. I knew then, with great certainty, that the child I had carried nine years before was a boy who someday would be all right.

I had pushed very hard for Danny to be removed from the respirator, against the doctors' wishes. When I saw other things stabilize--heart rate, blood pressure--I was sure there was no brain-stem damage. If there were, in fact, none, he could breathe on his own. I wanted to know that. They were, at that time, keeping him off the respirator at regular intervals.

When I went in shortly after seeing Danny running through green water, he was, in fact, receiving moisture and oxygen through a mask. I believe that night, somehow, our minds connected, and we both saw what we needed to keep going.

Danny came off the respirator completely about one month after the accident, and we moved all our acquired possessions up one floor to Moderate Care.

> Perseverance is more prevailing than violence; and
> many things which cannot be overcome when they are
> together, yield themselves up when taken little by little.
>
> --Plutarch

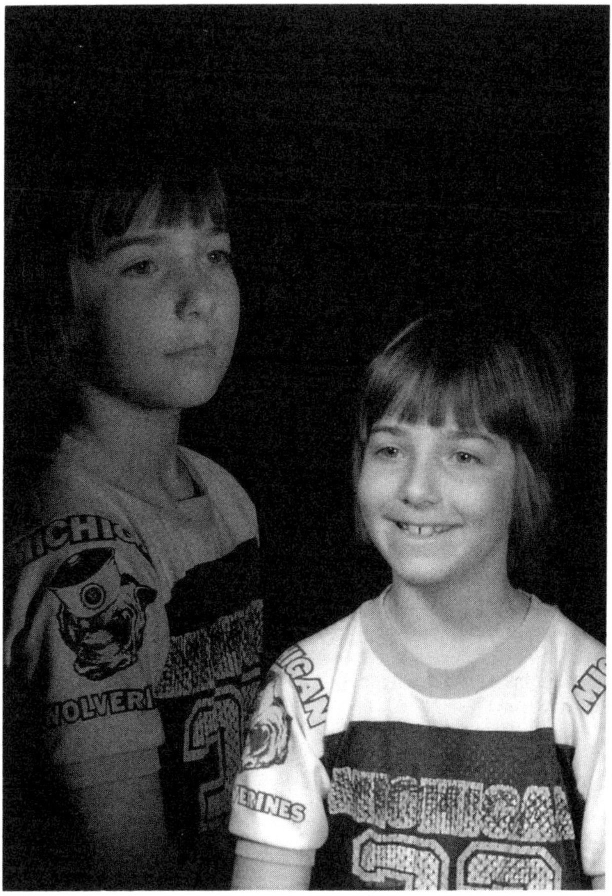

> Courage is the price that life exacts for granting peace. The soul that knows it not, knows no release from little things; knows not the livid loneliness of fear, nor mountain heights where bitter joy can hear the sound of wings.
>
> --Amelia Earhart

CHAPTER 3

Danny was wheeled in his bed out of Intensive Care, without the respirator, the chest tubes and the monitors. His leg still hung precariously from the traction bar, he was still intubated in case he had to be put back on the respirator, and had a new addition to his anatomy, a feeding tube.

The doctors, not wanting to continue putting tubes down Danny's throat for fear of infections and because they still believed he would remain in a persistent vegetative state for some time, had sought our signatures once again on another form to do a gastrostomy and a laryngectomy. Danny would be fed through a tube and could then be hooked up at a moment's notice to a respirator.

We signed the papers and waited anxiously while Danny was in surgery. When he returned, only the feeding tube had been inserted as his blood was not clotting, and they were afraid to cut again. Did we have any family history that would indicate a problem? Had this ever happened before? Perplexed, we could only wonder with the doctors as to why this occurred.

As a smaller child, Danny, not accident-prone but very active, often had cuts and scrapes. After several misadventures at age two, I was afraid to take him to a store--afraid someone might try to report me for child abuse! He loved to climb and would go as high as he could and then jump. His father had caught him at age three jumping from the rear of a six-foot high snowmobile trailer. I'm sure Danny had fun while it lasted, but the last jump included an additional jolt from his Dad.

All the bleeding in the past had always run the normal course. Why now? The report from the Lab: aspirin given Danny in the Emergency Room thinned the blood. They would have to wait to do the "trac". Danny never did have that surgery. Was it aspirin?

Moderate Care was a four-bed, ward-like room staffed by two nurses around the clock. Danny, although still unresponsive, was given injections of morphine every four hours for pain and to lessen agitation. Doug and I did a role reversal. Where his voice had been a calming factor in Intensive Care, I found if I sang Brahms Lullaby to Danny, he would rest. Also, the strain of carrying most of the weight for soothing Danny was beginning to show on Doug. He worried about the business, about our home and what the future held. Friends' efforts to support us nourished him less and less.

While we were still downstairs, friends Gerry and Helen Heiber had surprised us one night with a picnic in the waiting room. Steaks, baked potatoes, corn-on-the-cob and a bottle of wine were laid out over foot stools to not only our delight but others there. The nurses even joined in those few minutes of responding to life, which pulled us away from reacting to a near-death experience. At this point, even something like that would not have raised Doug from the pit of discouragement and despair in which he found himself.

We had found a cot and confiscated it for Doug to sleep on. One night when he sought solace in my arms, I rejected him. How could he think about having sex, and in a hospital waiting room. My son was in a coma, and he wanted sex. What kind of man was he? A normal man. As I look back now, it wasn't the sex, but the comfort from it he needed so desperately then. But I couldn't get past "me" far enough to see his needs.

Danny continued to improve physically but was still unresponsive. We held bed-side vigils. People still called daily, the cards and letters kept coming, but days came and went. We took turns leaving the hospital at this point, making a silent agreement that one of us would always be there.

With our daughters DeLyn and Denise, I went to the office after five, and we caught up backlogs of mail. We sent our policies, and I paid bills that had been forgotten for weeks. Out of sight, out of mind. I didn't care if creditors took it all. Things--our home, cars, credit rating--were really low on my priority list. But our insureds, many of whom had become more than clients over the years, they were our friends, drove us in our efforts to put service back to normal, or as close as we could, given the situation. So many of them were tolerant and stayed with us even through the delays. Their friendship and loyalty still leaves me without the words to thank them for all they gave us.

We took turns going home to shower and get clean clothes. Our neighbor, Bob Schnieder, whom we had lovingly called the "Sheriff of Meadow Lane" for years, watched our house and kept the yard mowed. How very blessed we were and didn't really realize it until weeks later.

We had woven for ourselves a cocoon of safety in that waiting room. Very competent nurses were taking care of Danny physically and trying to nourish us with information and support. The doctors kept their distance, and because the anger had to be directed somewhere, Doug and I both directed it at the physicians we felt were not telling us enough and were not doing what doctors are supposed to do. Didn't doctors make people better? Hadn't we always gone to the doctor for pills or a shot to make us well? Why weren't they fixing Danny? They weren't because Marcus Welby was a TV doctor, and,through the magic of television, patients woke up from comas, walked, talked and rejoined the human race right after the commercial break. We weren't living a television script; we were living life, and Danny wasn't waking up. Danny was the victim of what the medical community calls the "silent epidemic". Every year there will be 700,000 head injuries. Every year many of those will stay silent for a long time.

Doug had gone in to check on Danny and returned to the waiting room only to tell me to stay there 'til he returned. What I later found out was he had found blood coming out of Danny's mouth, and the nurse had called the doctor to come right away. He did not want me to see it, so one more time he went back in alone to confront fears that rip out your heart.

The doctor, one of the more abrasive ones with whom we had to deal, responded to the nurse's call. When his attitude, upon entering and leaving the unit, lit a spark in Doug, he chased the doctor down long hallways, but to our benefit, lost him in the maze of corridors. Doug returned and found that the movement of the bite block had been the culprit and the bleeding, although real, was not serious and was under control, once again by those special guardian angels in white, the nurses.

Not all the adventures or misadventures, if you will, were so serious or dire. Because of the traction rigging, Danny was moved about the hospital for tests while remaining in his bed. Four physicians came in to escort him elsewhere in the hospital complex and rolled the bed and all its attached equipment towards the door. The bed was too tall to pass through the door. In puzzlement, they turned the bed. It had come in through that door, why wouldn't it go out? They would have to dismantle the traction unit. The nurse smiled. No, they couldn't risk taking the pressure off the femur. The nurse smiled. How did the bed come into the unit? The nurse still smiled and let them walk around the bed in puzzlement, but only for a few more minutes before she asked them to push the bed back in its original position, plugged it in, then lowered the mattress so there was now plenty of clearance to go through the door.

We were only in Moderate Care a few days and were then moved up one more floor where Danny would now be put in a regular semi-private room. After five weeks of having a nurse right next to his bed, the idea of having him lay in a room all by himself and, unable to call for help frightened us. Our security was once again shaken by the change. We vowed that we would not allow him to be in that room alone for any extended period of time. This was reinforced when I came in and saw his tiny body lifting off the bed and found that the pain medication was an hour overdue. I visited the nurses station with less than a "please help him" attitude. We kept close watch from then on. The guarding also took its toll on our, by then, fragile nervous systems.

The Department of Physical Medicine, which had all along been sending in therapists to perform Range of Motion exercises to minimize muscle atrophy and contracture, stepped up their schedule. They also started planting the seeds of their rehab garden. What are you going to do when there is no longer a medical reason to keep Danny in the hospital? What did they mean no medical reason? Was he talking to me? Was he eating? Was he asking how long before he could play ball again? Of course he wasn't, and wasn't that medical reason enough to keep him? Didn't Marcus Welby keep patients in the hospital until they awoke and spoke? Didn't they fly in people from all over the world to this hospital?

And why were they talking about discharging Danny before he was my Danny again?

But they were, and they continued to do so. The bone, the femur, was healing to the point that the leg could be casted. Danny was breathing well on his own. He was taking nourishment through a tube which would remain as long as needed, and he was developing a regular waking/sleeping pattern. Although still unresponsive to stimuli, we should really consider where we were going to go from here.

July fourteenth was my birthday. Our daughter-in-law, Peggy, called and said we needed to get away from the hospital together and she would come and read and sing to Danny while we went out to celebrate, and our son, Doug, would take care of their two children while she was gone.

Reluctantly, we accepted the offer. Some birthday! The only present I wanted was to hear Danny say "Mom" and that wasn't happening. But go out we did. The Village Kitchen Restaurant, where we had eaten work-day lunches for years, seemed like the safest place to go. Familiar and friendly, it provided my 39th birthday dinner and gave my body and mind the first opportunity to relax it had had in weeks. The other nice thing was that the owner, who had shared Danny's growing-up with us, provided it free. Once again, we were cared for by the community and once again it didn't register until much later. How fortunate we were in this unfortunate adventure into unknowing and unknown.

After we left the restaurant, we stopped by the office to see what might take away the girls and I that weekend. In my office, which was not only an office but a place where everything that didn't fit elsewhere ended up, was a sofa. On that sofa that night, Doug and I made love in frenzied passion, not only yearning for the physical release, but the mental detachment, if only for a few minutes, from the pain that encircled our world. We returned to the hospital a little renewed by the experience and vowed to go on, to live, to fight another day.

And fight another day we did. For the next day, we were told that on the 16th, Danny's leg would be put in a cast and, as soon as the cast was dry, he was being discharged from the hospital. We could, the doctor said, put Danny in a nursing home, or take him home. There was no longer any medical reason for him to be hospitalized. They said he probably would remain in this vegetative state forever.

No medical reason? My son, who had been cared for by nurses, was now to be cared for by his mother who had no medical training, or go to a nursing home inhabited by people ten times his age? Damn the doctors. My old friend, adrenaline, kicked in. There had to be alternatives. Doors closed; new doors would open, or I'd break a window. Fear, anger, every survival instinct kicked into high gear.

I commandeered the pay phone. No one was calling out or taking a call until I found the third alternative. I called all the other hospitals in the area. None would accept a patient who was being discharged from another one. None had a program that would take Danny in this stage of coma. They had given us a copy of the Rancho Coma Scale, and when we read the description of the numbered levels, Doug had laughingly remarked that he thought he knew people who fit the description who were out walking around.

Our daughter, Denise, who was then working at Saline Community Hospital, a small community-based and supported facility which was connected to a nursing home, suggested that I go talk to Marilyn Koster, who was the head of their Speech Therapy Department, because other staff had spoken so highly of her.

Could I do that? Could I drive out of the parking structure and then past our house and then past that spot in the road where Danny's tiny, crumpled body had lain inaccessible to me? Could I drive past it? If it meant help for Danny, an alternative to the two options we had been given, I could do it. I could walk through fire, eat ground glass, WHATEVER it took. I went to Saline!

Marilyn saw me. She sat in one of the therapy rooms with me, gave me coffee and let me chain smoke as I poured out my tale of woe. This tiny woman nodded as I confessed my fears of inadequacy and then proceeded to tell me that often at home with familiar sounds, smells, surroundings, some patients respond better. People can come; there could be more stimulation; therapists could come to the house, and I was Danny's mother. I could care for him. Mothers can do that. Marilyn took away the fear and ignited a spark of determination that quickly flared into a full-blown fire. Danny was coming home! Coma or no coma, we'd do it. My attitude had just had, by the hope that Marilyn held out in front of me, an adjustment.

I heard a joke once about a farmer who had lost his wife of 40 years and with the insurance money had taken a trip to Las Vegas where he met and fell in love with a show girl. His friends were aghast that not only was it a short amount of time since his wife's death, but the show girl was forty years younger. When they talked to their friend, they voiced their concern and told him that the wedding night alone, given his age, could prove fatal. The old farmer just smiled and said, "Well, if she dies, she dies". Sometimes the best thing that can happen to us is to search for and listen to a fresh perspective. Marilyn had given me mine.

When I arrived back at the hospital, I told Doug we were taking Danny home. I called the insurance adjuster and told her I needed a hospital bed delivered to my house by the seventeenth, a wheelchair fitted to Danny, and that we were taking him home.

Marching to the nurses' station, I informed the nurses that they were to give me a crash course in Feeding Tube and Catheter 101, because I'd be taking care of Danny. God bless them, they all responded, and for two days they led me, over and over again, through the process. On Friday night after Danny was asleep, I left the hospital and drove home to start rearranging our downstairs to meet Danny's needs.

Our living room (which I'd never liked because it felt too formal)--after some things were moved out, others moved in and the rest rearranged--became Danny's new bedroom/sitting room. A big room, it could hold a number of people, and it was still in an area that could be closed off if need be.

I worked all night, returning to the hospital at five in the morning to see how many blue pads and swabs and those little things that help inflate your hospital bill I could talk the nurses out of. These ladies were sharp; they were one step ahead of me and had supplied what I hadn't even thought about, ready for me to take home with Danny.

Scared? Yes. Determined? Yes. Hopeful? More than ever. We'd show the doctors. It was good to take them home, "Marilyn said".

> Perhaps the most valuable result of an education is the ability to make yourself do the thing you have to do when it ought to be done, whether you like it or not; it is the first lesson that ought to be learned; and however early a man's training begins, it is probably the last lesson that he learns thoroughly.
>
> --Thomas Huxley

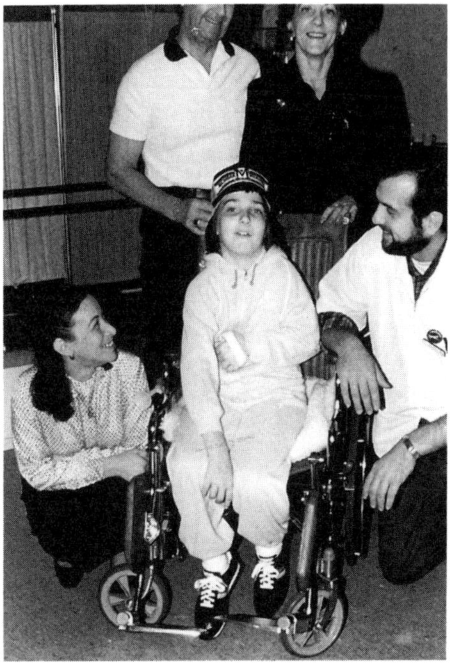

Dear Lord, bless this child and give him understanding.

Break down the barriers that are keeping him from grasping these skills, this knowledge. Stir and awaken his now dreaming mind.

Bless his books. Let your power and love work through them to excite and delight him so much that their message is clear and strong.

Bless his tools-his paper and pencils and crayons, so that they become lovely and sure, a source of joy to his hands.

Bless his teacher. Give her patience. Give her understanding. Give her the ability to guide him out of dark confusion into the light of comprehension and command.

Bless us, his mother and father. Help us to help him by being smarter ourselves. Halt our sometimes scolding tongues. Check our worry and concern. Fill us with so much pride in him - and so much faith in you - that he will feel it as a mighty force that encourages and moves him on.

For in you is all wisdom. And that wisdom is a part of our child.

I've Got to Talk to Somebody God
By: Marjorie Holmes

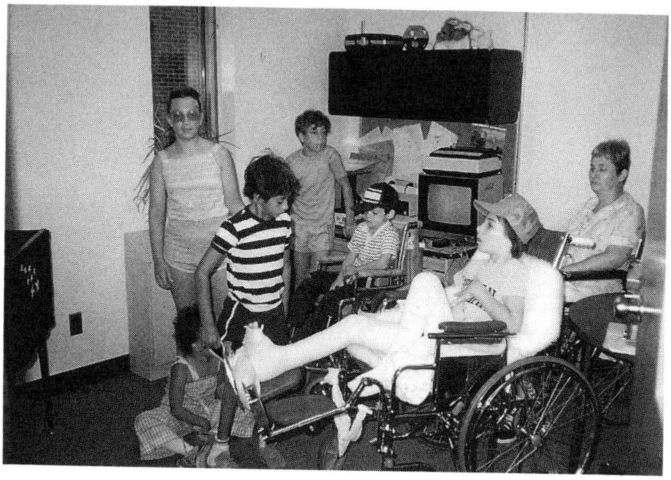

As a new parent when we hold the baby in our arms we make a covenant with that child to do all in our power to give him what we never had, what we think he should have, what we think is best for him. That covenant that we made to that small helpless, totally dependent baby is sometimes given to us twice in the lifetime of that same child when they sustain a head injury.

We're faced with starting all over. We must make a new covenant with that child. To give him all that's within our power to give. Remembering that we're the ones who must find resources, who must advocate, who must not accept what we're told but what we feel as the direction we take. We must find the strength and the courage to reach out into the same unknown that we ventured into as new parents. We did make it through once. Why not again?

> A personal commitment is one of life's high risk adventures. For when we commit ourselves to people we look into the future that is not going to be quite like the present, and we promise that we will be there, truly present, consistently and caringly, with people who may not be able to give us all we had expected from them. And the way we will make our commitment work is not by contract, not by force, but by the risky personal gift of trust.
>
> --Lewis B. Smedes

CHAPTER 4

Michigan No-Fault Auto, the goose that laid the golden egg for medical facilities in Michigan, was the primary insurance for Danny. All his medical bills for the rest of his life would be covered on our auto policy since he was struck as a pedestrian. That policy was paying for the rental of the equipment and would also pay for round-the-clock nursing care. As an insurance agent, I knew what was covered but let the nurse from the home health care company sent by the adjuster explain it to me anyway. No! I was not having a stranger take care of my son. I'd do it, and if I changed my mind, I'd call her. No, I didn't want ramps built or a new room on the house. We'd do it later, if necessary. Until then, they could leave me alone.

I never called, and it wasn't until a conversation years later that I found out the woman who was doing the scheduling for that company and with whom I now attended church, told me, "I knew when what you said was reported back, you'd never call". She was right on that as my now-dear friend, Janet, has been on other things which have impacted my life.

I watched over Danny during the day--charting times and amounts of cranberry juice, water and formula put through the tube. He was bathed and covered, the catheter was kept secured. Medical supplies purchased, suppositories administered on schedule and Colace, "liquid gold", by the price we paid per bottle, was given daily. I took over the half-bath downstairs, so I could always be within earshot and only went upstairs if someone was sitting near Danny.

Our neighbors, church members, and people within the community rallied, as well as those women who were with me as members of The Insurance Women of Washtenaw County. They coordinated schedules, and meals were brought in. My other children helped keep, or kept, the house clean and did most of the laundry. All I had to really do was take care of Danny. And take care of Danny I did, 24 hours a day. I slept sitting in a chair next to his bed. This person, who had slept a sleep like death since Danny had graduated from his crib, now awakened if his body twitched, or my hand with a lit cigarette fell into my lap and burned me, as well as the gown covering my leg. I still have several of them. At least I was consistent--they are all burned in the same spot. It was always me burned, never the chair, which could have caused even further problems. (When I was attending a Catholic girl's school as a teenager, even we Protestants were encouraged to say the rosary. We were told if we were saying it in bed and fell asleep, our guardian angel would finish it for us. My guardian angel kept me from starting a house fire and said all my prayers, because I was slowly exhausting myself, too tired to pray.)

Therapists from Saline Head Injury had been to the house to evaluate Danny, and we had set upon a schedule of taking him into the hospital daily for therapy. Doug jerry-rigged a ramp to get Danny into the van, and we took him ourselves, watching closely and trying very hard to do everything they suggested we do at home as carry-over.

Remember Sheriff Bob? He has a lovely wife, Carolyn, who is also a nurse, and she helped me with any number of questions and was always my safeguard if the feeding tube ever came out, which was the one caution I had received over and over from the nurses. Keep it dressed, don't let Danny pull it out. Carolyn helped me change the dressing around it and even managed to find a table just the right height for a TV set and Danny's Atari video game.

When Danny came home from the hospital, his right leg was casted to the hip, but the left leg moved freely. His right arm moved better than his left and his head stayed facing right. We couldn't bring, or keep, his head at mid-line. Marilyn suggested, because he would focus intently on the TV, that we move it one inch per day or so to the left.

This we did, and the head began to move. As Danny began to awaken from the coma, his left side began drawing up. The heel of his left foot drew closer and closer to his butt. I would pull the leg back and massage the muscles, but it finally became an impossibility to straighten the leg. The left arm drew up as in a sling, and the fingers bent out backwards. He was awakening, but physically we were going backwards. Therapists made splints.

Danny still couldn't talk or take food by mouth except for the very soft, or if we made it the consistency of baby food, as he would not chew. His tenth birthday came and went. He swears he remembers it, but he doesn't. His memory before the accident was now partially intact. Although he couldn't talk, he could point to his eye, his heart and the person he intended it for--signing "I love you". The tears that brought when I finally realized what he was doing!

Doug had promised Danny in the hospital that as soon as he woke up, he would give him his wish that his Daddy would quit smoking. One day, sitting next to Danny, Doug lit up a cigarette. Tears welled up in Danny's eyes. Doug threw away the cigarettes.

Danny wanted pizza; that's all he thought about from every indication. (While in therapy at Saline Hospital, the therapists, who knew he liked pizza, would ask him if he would like to have pizza. His eyes would get big and he would smile, confirming he did indeed want it.) He couldn't have it because he wouldn't chew, and the therapists puzzled over what to do to get that response to kick in. "Did Danny like bubble gum?" Did Danny like bubble gum?! He was seldom without it! What respectable baseball pitcher would be seen not chewing. Since tobacco was out of the question, bubble gum was the next best thing. So, wrapped in gauze, a string tied around it, bubble gum was put in Danny's mouth. We waited. No movement. Waited longer. Sugar must be getting on his tongue and it was. That taste kicked in a memory, and he started chewing. It was time to order the pizza.

Danny's vocal chords, held apart for so long while he was intubated, needed to be coaxed now into making sound, and there were things Danny wanted to say. He worked on a special machine where every sound registered, and he blew water from one tube to the other. When National Public Radio did a program on the Saline Head Injury program, Danny croaked into the phone, and his father and I talked to the interviewer. We were on our way. Danny wanted to talk and set about doing just that.

Now that he could chew and was able to take nourishment by mouth, the doctor agreed to remove the feeding tube. We took Danny in and were relieved to finally be rid of that little ugly piece of brown rubber that we had moved so delicately for weeks, afraid it would fall out. However, when the doctor tried to slip it out, it wouldn't budge. She pulled harder and short of putting her foot on his chest, pulled yet harder. It came out. A mushroom-shaped end the size of a quarter came out through a hole about the size of a very narrow pencil! The doctor, although I'm sure had been pleased by Danny's speech progress, was not happy with what then came out of his mouth. Danny grabbed the tube from her hand and threw it against the wall! All those days of worrying that the tube would come out, handling it like it was a Ming vase had all been unnecessary; but it was out, we'd made one more step. He might be a cauliflower, but this vegetable could talk, could eat, and now we'd go on.

The first part of August, Doug had gone back to work. He had spent 25 years building this business, and he was getting concerned about the service to the people who had become part of his life over those years. He was also realistically concerned over our income. We had no idea how much our financial contribution to Danny's recovery and lifetime care might be.

By the end of August, the office was still not running smoothly and the backlog caused more anxiety for this perfectionist husband of mine. The fact our summer employee was leaving for college really threw Doug into a tailspin. One night he came home from the office and as we talked, he put his head in his hands and said, "If you can't get it straightened out, I'm going in and set a match to it". Super-wife to the rescue! Doug would stay home, take Danny to therapy. I would go in, run the office, get it organized. Hire staff, take care of the housework and laundry (those things at night), spend time with Danny, serve as President of Insurance Women and complete my Accredited Advisor in Insurance program. I could do that. No problem.

DeLyn and Denise jumped in with both feet. The young lady we hired was quick and capable. Within two weeks, the office, although not producing new business, was at least caught up. Daughters, who had not only been around the business all their lives but had each worked for us in the past, helped train.

I sent out appreciation letters, hundreds, and signed each one. As I addressed the envelopes and saw familiar names, those (so many) who took time to embrace us in our time of need through cards, phone calls and prayers, became even more special. It certainly had been worth our time and effort, even though some of it was given grudgingly. The old axiom, "What goes around, comes around", or, "As you sow, so shall you reap", certainly was true and took on even deeper meaning.

Therapy was now scheduled for twice a day. Danny would go in the morning, come home for lunch and an hour's rest and then return. After dinner, we'd do the repetitive range-of-motion exercises, plus new ones designed to bring strength back to weakened muscles, much needed if we were going to get Danny back on his feet. They rolled him around on a big ball in therapy to help with balance, and we started holding him upright with support to keep weight off the cast.

I still slept in the room with Danny on a twin bed next to him but no longer with my hand on him to awaken at a movement. He could now let me know if he needed something. The catheter had been replaced by a urinal, much to Danny's delight. He thought it was pretty neat to not have to get up.

Doug still slept alone in the king-size bed we'd shared for years. I couldn't go up there and leave Danny alone. But in September, I did sneak away a couple of times to be held in the comfort of arms that had rescued me from the world for years. Maybe our lives would someday be put back together as in a jig-saw puzzle; when each new piece filled that gaping hole, we were closer to being a whole family again. But in that jig-saw puzzle, the pieces must go where they belong, or the whole thing is thrown off.

We had settled into a routine, and I ran on a finely tuned schedule. I had a daily planner where therapists' appointments, meetings, classes, household chores, errands, Doug's schedule and mine were down to ten minutes, one way or the other. Danny also had to fit into this. A homebound teacher provided by the school district for those children who could not go to school. We wanted to try and keep Danny up with the children he had started school with. I could find time to help with homework, too.

October came, and I encouraged Doug to plan his annual treks to the north woods for archery (deer) season. He had been going for years, and I knew he needed to get away, to go where maybe if he couldn't see all the paraphernalia that meant illness, he could find solace and renewed strength. Me, I didn't need that. I was strong! Wanting to go, but torn between that and the feeling of dumping all the responsibility on me, "the spouse guilt syndrome", he couldn't make a decision. Then he did. I could go with him and Danny, still in a cast, still in a wheelchair; and we could entertain ourselves in a pick-up truck camper while he was out hunting.

Never being one to mince words, the words that shot out of my mouth at that suggestion touched off the fuse for the most explosive argument we'd had since Danny was injured. Doug went to work; I left him a note that said, "You'd better start thinking about what you're going to do when Danny is well, because I'm out of here".

When Doug came home from the office, I was dressed and ready to leave. The Insurance Women were doing a fashion show to raise funds for Cystic Fibrosis that evening, and, as the President I was to present the check to the Cystic Fibrosis Chapter President. As I went out the door, Danny called me back. On his bedstand was some change and a dollar bill. One of the things Marilyn had learned as Danny's reason returned was that he responded well to bribery. Money meant he could go to the hospital gift shop to get candy or gum. He also liked the attention that the volunteers who operated the gift shop gave him. And I appreciated this, as now the encouragement they offered him, as well as the cheering of his progress, kept him going.

Danny reached over and got the dollar. "Mom, please give this to Cystic Fibrosis. Those kids need it more than I do." Tears that I was becoming more familiar with stung my eyes as I hugged this very special son of mine. He truly had been sent by angels.

I was leaving earlier than necessary because I was still smarting from the argument with Doug that morning. He'd had the gall to tell me I was selfish. Selfish because I wouldn't keep Danny in a truck camper for the weekend while he was out hunting. Selfish because that was his solution to going hunting and not having to feel guilty. How dare he! Selfish! Was I selfish as I cared for Danny? Wasn't it me who rubbed those contracting limbs all night while he slept? Wasn't it me who went to work when he couldn't handle it? Wasn't it me who monitored

Danny's therapies? Selfish! How dare he, I thought, as I pulled into the shopping center.

Credit cards at the ready, I was going to spend some money. That would make me feel better and one of the more expensive stores would be better yet. As I walked in the door, the jewelry counter was straight ahead. Although buying jewelry had not been my intention, I started looking. Rings, diamond rings. Yes, that would be good. A big diamond cocktail ring. Yes, that would be REALLY good. The card limit was high enough, and we'd had it for years. They'd raise the limit, if necessary. I bought a ring, not a cheap one, that sparkled on my finger as I entered the hotel that was hosting the fashion show and, walked into the room with my ring, in my business suit, in my most presidential manner.

There were a few comments on my ring, and I just said, "Oh, that's my selfish ring", without offering an explanation. When it came time to present the check to the Cystic Fibrosis President, a man I'd worked with for three years, I explained the check and the one dollar bill, leaving not a dry eye in the room, including mine. The ring sparkled on my finger.

When I got home much later than usual that night and with several glasses of wine inside me, Doug was waiting up. We had to talk. He was sorry. How fortunate I was and am to have a man who is not afraid to say that, because he married a woman who very rarely says that. If it comes out of my mouth, I've always figured I meant to say it, and I'm not sorry I said it!

We held each other; I cried some more, and we vowed to work something out. The ring sparked on my finger, and I didn't tell Doug about buying it. That was my selfish ring, and he didn't need to know about it and wouldn't for eight years.

The compromise we arrived at was that he would go hunting. I would get up early on Saturday, drive Danny up to Houghton Lake, spend the day, and we'd come home that evening if Danny wanted; otherwise, he and I would stay in a motel in town. Our older son, David, would ride with us in case there was car trouble, so Danny would not be left alone.

Doug went hunting. When we got there on Saturday, he looked refreshed and for the first couple of hours Danny enjoyed the woods. It didn't take long for him to tire of the chair. No longer could he run through the woods. The damage done to the optic nerve which affected one eye and his vision took the fun out of target practice. The weather, not bad, was also not good. He wanted to go home.

A trip into Houghton Lake and fortified for the return trip by a banana split, we came home, while Dad stayed to hunt and get recharged by another day. Danny cried that night. He wanted to walk again. With only the guts and determination an unknowing parent can have, I promised him he'd walk--we'd find a way.

Two weeks later, the x-ray showed that the bone had mended and was reinforced by additional calcification. The cast could come off. Back to the rooms just down the hall from the hospital Emergency Room where we had waited months earlier, we took Danny to have the cast cut off. There we found a laughing, friendly technician who remembered Danny from that fateful day and shared with us his joy in seeing Danny doing so well. He cut the cast off amidst Danny's exhortation, "Don't cut my leg", and the hairy, withered right leg emerged. The cast looked better than what had been exposed, but Danny wanted to walk. We'd walk!

Before we left the hospital, we walked back through the familiar halls to the Intensive Care Unit. We wanted to show off this young man who doctors had said would never do anything. We were fortunate to find on duty the pretty little nurse who had stood her vigil over Danny that first night, not wanting to return the second because she didn't think he'd make it. But return she did, to care for Danny and for us, and we were returning to show her what her watch/care had produced. What a joy it was for all of us to leave that floor this time with a brighter future ahead. Danny would come back; Danny would be a functioning person. After all, hadn't "Marilyn said".

A lot of work and a lot of pain lay ahead for Danny. The left leg had to straighten out. The right leg, weakened by lack of use for those four months, had to be strengthened. Danny's physical therapist, who now 10-year-old Danny was developing a crush on, tested his mettle.

Danny had started his introduction to standing on an incline table. The first experience had not been a happy one but getting him up often had gotten his head used to the different blood supply; and although he was no longer dizzy, balance eluded him. He worked on the exercises, walked up and down the parallel bars, and pride in each accomplishment glowed on his face.

> Nothing in the world can take the place of persistence. Talent will not; nothing is more common than unsuccessful men with talent.
>
> Genius will not; unrewarded genius is almost a proverb. Education will not; the world is full of educated derelicts. Patience and determination alone are important.
>
> --Calvin Coolidge

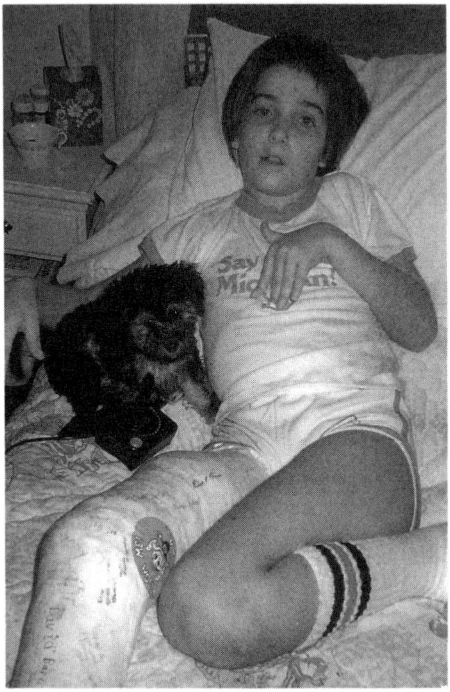

One of the most difficult things everyone has to learn is that for your entire life you must keep fighting and adjusting if you hope to survive. No matter who you are or what your position, you must keep fighting for whatever it is you desire to achieve.

If someone is not aware of this contest and expects otherwise, then constant disappointment occurs. People who fail sometimes do not realize that the simple answer to everyday achievement is to keep fighting.

Health, happiness and success depend upon the fighting spirit of each person. The big thing is not what happens to us in life but what we do about what happens to us.

George H. Allen

It is one of the most beautiful compensations of this life that no man can sincerely try to help another without helping himself.

--Emerson

CHAPTER 5

Knowing our family needed to get back to church, I had told the Pastor of the church (situated on the road where Danny had been hit) that as soon as Danny could get around, we'd be there. In November, just before Thanksgiving, we attended a Sunday service and were greeted warmly by Danny's fourth-grade teacher, friends from Little League and those parishioners who had helped pray us through. We supported Danny as he walked. We were in church, surrounded by not only the love of that congregation but God's love. It felt good to be back in church; I felt at home.

As we filed out after services and shook hands with Pastor Siegel, Danny tugged on my arm. "I want to show him I can walk, Mom. All by myself, Mom." By now, I'd learned to not let my fears get in between Danny and one of his goals, so turning around, I released him and watched him take six faltering steps--the most at any one time until that day--into the waiting arms of Pastor Siegel. My eyes weren't the only ones that filled with tears that day. I wondered if Danny would continue to keep me acquainted with tears that I had always before seen as a sign of weakness. Big girls didn't cry, or so I had come to believe and live my life by, until I had been blessed with this child, by the angels.

When Danny was little and had asked where he came from, I had responded by saying, "from the angels", and he accepted that. When in the first grade he got his first taste of sex education, he taunted his older brother by saying, "You came from Mom's tummy, but I came from the angels". By now he knew the real story, but I'm not sure yet that his essence, the part of us that can't be seen or touched, the part that makes him so uniquely Danny, wasn't touched by one.

By Christmas, Danny was able to traverse his way the length of our family room. We could get him up and down stairs; he could sleep in his old room, his bed. The hospital bed could go, but the wheelchair had to remain for long distances.

In January, Danny's homebound teacher, who had brightened all our days since September, felt Danny should be reintegrated to his classroom. She could work with him there and school could wrap around his therapy, and everything could be coordinated so Danny could have some socializing, classwork and therapy. She went before us and talked to Danny's classmates about what to expect. I found myself sitting in the teacher's lounge two hours every morning while Danny was in the classroom, being hovered over by all the kids who were determined to look out for him. Danny was comfortable in that element much more than I.

I remembered David and recalled cutting remarks from my own grade school peers. I didn't want Danny hurt, but Danny was holding his own. His verbal skills, now good and his sense of humor, held him in good stead. This child of mine, the one with brain damage, my little cauliflower, was still handling all of this better than Mom.

Therapy was going well. We really didn't see the plateaus they had warned us about. We'd level off, and then all of a sudden there would be a breakthrough. One day Danny was balking at doing the required task in Speech. Marilyn, resorting back to bribery, said to Danny, "If you will finish the one thing, there is a dollar on my desk and you can have it to go to the gift shop". Undaunted, Danny, whose quick wit was continuing to emerge, said, "Why don't you give me five and call me cured?" Needless-to-say for days around the therapy unit, people were slapping hands and saying, "Give me five and call me cured".

Summer came, along with Little League season. How Danny mourned the fact he couldn't play baseball but was still determined that someday he would once again hit those home runs that had gotten him newspaper coverage and slaps on the back from coaches previously.

I came from a small farm community and left it as soon as I was old enough to hit the road. I had always hated that town and felt the minds of the inhabitants were as small or smaller than the town. Unlike the community of my childhood, the small German farm community we found ourselves in, a bedroom community to the much larger town where we worked, responded to our family and Danny.

The town barber had come out to the house to cut Danny's hair early on. The dental hygienist had come to clean his teeth. There were food, calls, cards, as well as the response of the school system to try and accommodate Danny's needs as well as the response from local business. Once when I wanted to send pizzas and pop over to the school for the last day of fifth grade, the manager of the local Pizza Hut came in early, made 40 individual pan pizzas and had them ready. He even took a check which was against policy because I was "Danny's Mom". That soon became my new recognition factor. I was no longer "Doug's wife"; I was "Danny's Mom".

The Little League coaches responded the same way. Danny was on a team. Back on the pitcher's mound with another player standing really close to field those balls that Danny's left arm could not always be depended upon to catch. What if he got hurt out there? Well, what if he did. Boys got hurt on ball fields. If Danny were going to be hurt again, wasn't it better if he were hurt doing a normal boy's activity? Wasn't that pain better than those hours of stretches he had endured with clenched teeth and teary eyes? Our concerns didn't matter, Danny was to have that chance. We didn't know then that it would be the last summer Danny would be on a real team on a ball diamond, but he at least had that year.

The hometown newspaper which had followed Danny's progress once again sent a reporter to take a picture of Danny on the mound. We had stopped being alone when we brought Danny home from the hospital. The whole town cheered Danny's progress. How fortunate we felt once again that as long as this tragedy had to happen, two doctors from the children's hospital happened to be right behind the van that hit him. We were also close to an excellent trauma center--not only because the much-needed life-saving physicians were only minutes away, but unlike many families who sat waiting with us which had come from miles away to seek help for their children, our home was less than fifteen minutes away. Therapy was almost within walking distance, and the community was small enough that we didn't get lost. People knew Danny and continued to cheer his progress.

As I sat in church on Sunday mornings, I couldn't help but say, "Thank you, God". But as in everyone's life, there were times when I didn't say that.

The left side was still a problem. Although Danny could use his left hand fairly well, the arm didn't move properly at the shoulder; the left leg rotated out at the hip and his left foot turned out in duck fashion. His short-term memory, although improving, was still affected; he couldn't get a handle on a lot of the school work.

When Danny first emerged from his coma and for the first few months, he'd ask if we could have pizza. I'd say, "Sure". He'd then ask if we could get hamburgers. I'd say, "Sure". Then, "Could I go play video games?" "Sure, Danny". I knew it would change in a few minutes, so it was easy to agree because he'd forget. It was with mixed emotions that I got trapped into something I had not intended when he did remember and said to me, "Mom, you said", and I had. We quit being so quick to say, "Sure, Danny", right there and then.

This was improvement, Danny was getting better. But occasionally, as I saw something cut Danny to the quick, or we would not move as fast as I thought we should, I would rail at God. Often out in our front yard with tears in my eyes and a lump in my throat, I would say, "Quit growing me, quit growing us. We don't need anymore growing by overcoming hardships and life's challenges. You can touch him and heal him. Just do it. Do it now. I've had enough. Danny's had enough." Our ways are not always God's ways, the pastor says on Sunday morning. Well, no kidding. I'm tired of this. I want my son back. He saved his life--for this? To always be confronted with things he can't do? Well, thank you, God. Thanks for nothing!

But those things, those feelings, although intense, were fleeting; and I would move one more step forward. Or someone would come into our lives that held out a promise, and I would say, "Thank you, God," hoping his promise to love me and forgive me and hold this mother, "Danny's Mom", in his arms while she cried, would get us through the days ahead.

As children bring, in tears, their broken toys for us to mend, I gave my broken dreams to God because He was my friend.

But then instead of leaving him in peace to work alone, I hung around and tried to help with ideas of my own.

I finally snatched them back and cried, "How can you be so slow?"

"My child," He said, "I want to help, but first you must let go."

--Author Unknown

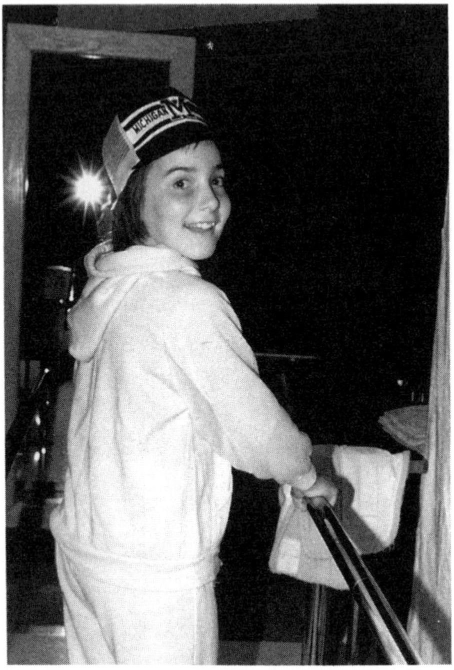

In the beginning
God created the heaven
and the earth.

And the earth was
without form and void:
and darkness was upon
the face of the deep.
And the spirit of God
moved upon the face
of the waters.

And God said,
Let there be light:
and there was light.

Genesis 1:1-3

Judaism, Hinduism, Buddhism, and Christianity, Islam, all speak of the light. Sometimes it comes to us in the face and through the love and the courage of a child.

Judith Wharton

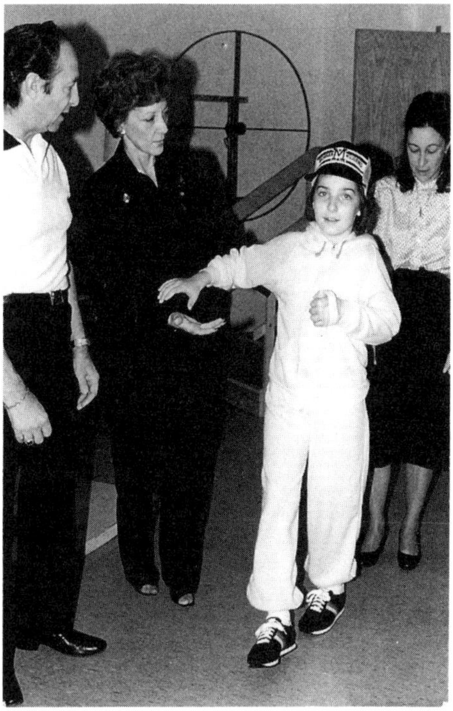

Ecclesiastes 4:9-12

Two are better than one because they have a good return for if either of them falls, the other one will lift up his companion.

But woe to the one who falls when there is not another to lift him up. Furthermore, if two lie down together they keep warm, but how can one be warm alone?

And if one can overpower him who is alone, two can resist him. A cord of three strands is not quickly torn apart.

Danny was the piece of cord that contained a fiber stronger than steel, and he helped the fabric which was his parents hold together.

> People are always blaming their circumstances for what they are. I don't believe in circumstances. The people who get on in this world are the people who get up and look for the circumstances they want, and, if they can't find them, make them.
>
> --George Bernard Shaw

CHAPTER 6

We were into our second year. The wheelchair long since returned to the rental company. Danny walking with that same awkward gait, arm still drawing up and more so when he was intent upon using his right hand and arm. It was time to get innovative. Time to wrap bubble gum in gauze again.

As we entered into our second year, Danny was better. But the first son that I had asked God to spare went through his senior year of high school virtually unnoticed. We had been so wrapped up in Danny that David was often left to fend for himself. We didn't even realize how much more we could have done to help him have the best year ever. He would from now on pass into adulthood, and we'd missed the whole last year. I threw myself into graduation party arrangements. This also helped me get through June 10th with hardly an awareness of what day it was. It didn't work that way for Doug, but he made it through.

Before Danny was born, I had had, for the sake of naming it, an identify crisis. I had gone through several sessions with a pastor/counselor using hypnosis, and I had liked the results in me. I also had read a number of things on the subconscious mind. I wondered, if we tapped into Danny's subconscious--through hypnosis--could we bypass the areas of damage, could we train another area of the brain to take over? I called the now-retired minister. What did he think; was there a chance?

"There's always a chance, Sue," was all he'd say, so I kept the phone lines busy.

A client, a psychiatrist, gave me the name of a psychologist that used hypnosis. I called him. He'd see Danny. We began years 2, 3, and 4. Through weeks of hypno-therapy and biofeedback training, the arm relaxed and was at Danny's side. Through concentration, he could isolate muscles that would move pictures on a television screen. We'd made some progress but not a hundred percent, because there was still functional deficits. Danny's therapist located a sports medicine clinic that had a computer-operated exercise machine. We took Danny there to work on the arm and leg. One more step. Danny could walk normally on the treadmill, but we could get no carryover. He could relax his arm, but it would begin to draw up when he was concentrating on something else.

A new sports medicine clinic opened forty miles away. I took Danny there three days a week. The rapport he established with the therapist/owner, as well as state of the art equipment, got Danny enthused about physical therapy again and strengthened weakened areas, but we couldn't overcome the muscles that were tight and kept so by the brain.

New doctor on Cape Cod. He had had success in doing alcohol blocks in muscles. Maybe that would work. We flew to Boston, rented a car, and drove to the Cape, had Danny evaluated and returned home that evening. The one thing that we had always felt important and continued to feel was that Danny's therapy and school schedule be strictly adhered to. He had to be really ill to stay home. "Mom, I'm tired" never worked. We were all tired, but I was scared. Scared if we backed off even a little, Danny might want a little more and then a little more.

Soon after we had started going to church again, a guest minister told the story of a nasty little boy who spent his time catching the rather tiny little birds which lived near his home. They were small enough so that he could completely hide one in his hands. After catching one, he would go up to someone and telling them he had a bird in his hand and asked them to guess if the bird were alive or dead. If they guessed that the bird was dead, he would open his hand, and the bird would fly away. If they said the bird was alive, he would squeeze his hands together and, needless to say, the little bird did not fly away. One day, he was walking down the street with a tiny bird clenched in his fist, when he saw an old woman approaching. She was stooped and her hand wiggled at the top of a cane. He ran up to her and asked her to guess, was the bird alive or dead. She looked at him for a moment and then said, "It seems to me the future is in your hands."

That's the way I felt. The direction for Danny, his future, lay in my hands, and I couldn't lighten up. I didn't want to ever get so comfortable with the status quo that I quit searching for another technique that would take Danny one step closer to complete wellness. I couldn't get too comfortable and then fail to take a risk. Danny had a lifetime ahead of him, and that lifetime had to have the highest quality possible. I had to learn to open my hand and let him fly.

The doctor on the Cape was willing to give it a try. Danny's left shoulder, which had frozen before and had to be broken free under anesthetic, had frozen again. He would take care of that while Danny was in the operating room. We were to make arrangements to come back to the Cape and be prepared to stay a week, if necessary. We made the arrangements. A month later, they were rolling Danny into the operating room.

The doctor requested permission from the OR to cut the tendon in Danny's arm to give it more opportunity to move. We said okay. It was summer on the Cape, and the census of the hospital was down. Our son had a whole wing to himself and nothing better to do than entertain the round-the-clock nurses. That first afternoon, with some of the alcohol having gotten into his system, he was ready to party. What he wasn't ready for was being sick and his first experience with a hangover. I remember telling Doug, "Maybe he'll never want to drink if he thinks this is what will follow." After three days, we installed Danny in the back seat for the long drive back to Michigan. I knew we'd found the answer to Danny's mobility problem. Hadn't I searched for a long time; wasn't it time for us to be done with the long therapy hours, and for Danny to have a normal kid schedule? It was by our calendar but not by life's. Although there had been some improvement in the arm and leg, the two outside fingers and the side of his hand were numb. We had to watch now to be sure he didn't hurt them and not notice. The loss of sensation threw Danny off, he had to work on walking again. Although it loosened the muscle tone, there was no real change in his walk or his ability to use his left hand. Well, wasn't year three just wonderful?

I took on even more projects away from home to keep me busy. I kept a frantic pace. I would take Danny to school, go to the office, leave to pick him up, and we'd go to therapy. I took work with me so I could continue to keep an eye on what was going on and try to pick up any bit of information I could about what we could try next.

Late in our first year we had become involved in a Head Injury support group. With us now going into the third year, I could take on another committee, I could do a newsletter, and I could help find speakers. I had time in my day to think, and I still didn't want to. Must keep busy.

The family support group was an escape to a safe haven one night once a month. A small group that gave each other permission to be unshakable, democratic, and comforting. It also meant we gave others permission to hold us accountable. I very much needed to hear that others had survived the pain that I carried with me daily. I needed information; I needed to hear and to share experiences. But the most important thing I needed then, but didn't know right away, was to learn that I could and it would be okay to someday laugh again. How fortunate I was to be in a group that had as one of its members the Don Rickles of Head Injury humor. She told us stories. Of the neurosurgeon who, upon looking at her comatose son, shook his head and said, "What a shame, he was such a handsome young man." Hardly able to contain herself with the surgeon's obvious demonstration of compassion, she responded, "Would it have been better if he'd been ugly?" These kinds of stories fed into our displaced anger at the doctors who had saved our children's lives. They were a safe scapegoat. We didn't plan on seeing them again, and we all walked carefully in the other areas of our lives.

Marriages made tenuous by the crisis that befell us, we all knew the statistics on how many did not survive a head injury; we had to strive to keep ours intact. She told of her husband who snored and how he would hold his breath as she waited for the sound to come. One night, when it seemed longer than usual, she hit him in the chest and said, "Don't you die on me and leave me alone to handle this." Imagine being awaken that way. Yes, many of us were afraid of that, too. Sometimes all I wanted was Doug to be quiet and stay out of my way. Other nights I would look over at the man sleeping beside me and be ever so thankful that he was there. How could I handle this all alone, even though "I knew" I was doing all the work, if I didn't have the support his love gave me? Also, Danny, as he had since he first said the word "Daddy", adored his father and worked hard, not for my approval but for Dad's.

The stress and strain of coping with the changed family unit often brings on other major life events. My teacher of humor found her husband in the hospital Cardiac Unit. Heart attack. How could he? As she retold the story of her asking him the same question, "How could you do this to me? You did it on purpose so I'd have to deal with this alone. You're taking the easy way out. How dare you." The animation, the tone of voice, our meeting room roared with the Emergency room humor that often gets so many through. We were laughing at what was one of the things we all feared most, being alone. But it was okay to laugh. Hadn't we found out that even though the fear didn't go away that laughter was good for each of us? The medical community was now studying the effects of chemicals released by the brain during laughter to see if it was truly beneficial to human health and well being. The medical community was doing a study on something our little group already knew. That even though it did not always seem appropriate, it helped us survive.

Danny maintained. He gave everything his best. He worked on his school work; he did the therapy projects, and longed to play baseball. I was not going to tell him he probably would never play. How did I know that? Look what he had accomplished so far. Hadn't I fired a doctor who the year before had told me I had to tell Danny that there would be things he could never do because he was handicapped? After I'd left his office in tears, I had to eat dirt and go back to the original rehab physician that I'd left for similar reasons. But she was amazed with Danny's progress and was willing to work with me and did write the orders for the nontraditional therapies that we had been trying. Danny was doing much better mentally with only some memory problem, and his always quick wit and sense of humor not only remained but it blossomed even more.

One day while he was at therapy, he sat down in an empty wheelchair belonging to another little boy, also in therapy. The hospital chaplin, who never failed to talk to Danny and encourage his progress, passed by the therapy room. When he saw Danny in a wheelchair again, real concern caused him to retrace his steps.

To his question of, "What happened, Danny?", Danny responded with "Didn't you hear, I've had a relapse and I'm back in a chair."

The Reverend shook his head and said how "sorry he was to hear that." Everyone else in the waiting room held their breaths, wondering what would come next.

Danny then proceeded to tell the Reverend that "he just knew if he put his hand on the front of his head and said a prayer, it would help."

The poor, unsuspecting Man of the Cloth did just that. After he had said "Amen" and removed his hand, Danny arose from the chair, arms in the air, and said, "Praise the Lord, I've been healed." The poor, unsuspecting Reverend had just gotten a first-hand view of the humor of this son of mine. The receptionist said his face was so red--given his age, she was afraid he'd have a heart attack.

The next day Danny had to seek out the Reverend and apologize. But once again, the theme in the therapy department had been set by Danny. "Praise the Lord, I've been healed." His humor, not always that shocking, served him well, and his smiles and cooperative manner served him well in his relationships. It was hard for him to have much social life because of the grueling schedule, but we did take him on one vacation a year, and he got to just "veg out" during the Christmas break.

As an insurance agent, Doug qualified for the Company's promotional trips every year, so Danny went to Germany, Hawaii, Bermuda, and Acapulco. We had to listen to the older kids lament the fact we'd never taken them. Once we could afford to put four or five on an airplane with us, we couldn't have. College and dental work took a lot of money for a long time, and just feeding four teenagers wasn't cheap. When the two younger girls left home at almost the same time, our electric bill dropped fifty dollars a month, and they had expected a trip, too? We took Danny not only because we could better afford it, but because we didn't want to leave him home where anything might happen. Fear of losing him still often made our decisions for us.

Puberty, the cracking voice, the noticing of girls, the yearning for independence hit Danny like a Mack truck. Now, as a teenager, he wanted more freedom. What kind of freedom? To be left home alone for awhile. All by himself. What was the matter with us? Why did someone always have to be there? Didn't we know he could take care of himself? Why didn't we just go out and leave him alone? He could take care of the house. He was a teenager, after all. Believing that what he said did have merit, we were still uncomfortable leaving to go somewhere that maybe we couldn't be reached. Taking care of Danny and Danny's needs had become such a way of life, we struggled very hard even with the thought of change. We were locked into the status quo that we'd feared for Danny. Danny had become much like the starfish washed upon the beach--he needed help. As parents, we needed to be like the man who walked along the beach picking them up and throwing them back into the water. When asked why he was doing this--because they probably would only wash up to lay there again, what difference could he make--he threw one out and responded, "I'm making a difference to this one." We needed to throw the starfish into the water, needed to give the little bird a nudge from the nest. We'd do even what birds know they have to do, let go.

We went out for coffee; we went into the office at night; we eventually over time were gone long enough to see a movie. Each time we returned to Danny's statement, "See, I can be alone."

We were learning more from this child who had already, through his courage and determination, taught us so much. We even managed that year to hire someone to come in, take Danny to school and therapy, and Doug and I spent four days alone at a company convention in Toronto. Maybe we were going to be okay. Maybe there would be a life for us again. Maybe.

Our other children married and divorced, had children, and bought first homes. Our family grew and life went on. We had reached another plateau. Danny was doing well on the interpersonal skills, managing the homework with help, growing in independence, but the physical problems still persisted. The odd gait, the left hand and arm still frustrated Danny's physical therapist. With necessity often being the mother of invention, she pulled from her own experience with the Martial Arts and not only convinced the hospital to underwrite the program but convinced a local Tae Kwon Do instructor that they could have a class, and she would help. There were five head-injured patients plus two aides in the first class. Danny, who had been a big fan of Kungfu on TV when he was little, running around in a robe and yelling "Hi Ya!" at two and three, was really excited about this program. Outfitted in their white tobacs and white belts, they were an odd blend of capabilities as they set off towards a new goal . . . yellow belt.

They were going to learn kicks and punches, they were going to break boards. One mother asked me if I wasn't afraid of Danny breaking his hand. As with the baseball, I responded, "At least he'll break it doing something normal." Bones break; bones heal. A broken bone no longer wrapped me in fear. Hadn't the benchmark for fear already been established for me with Danny's head injury? Nothing ever again could ever be that bad. I had something to measure every other even in my life against. If it weren't an injury to the head, we'd get through it.

Danny still had some balance problems. We had had surgery on the optic nerve that had caused his left eye to look at you at an odd angle. The double vision had been corrected, but some depth perception problems would probably remain to be compensated for. Our determined son had ridden his bike up and down the driveway and fallen an equal number of times until his body had kicked in with its own compensatory skills, which now allowed him to ride anywhere he wanted. But now he must balance on one foot--make turns, lift the leg to kick and not tip over. The left arm, which sometimes had a will of its own, needed to block and to punch. Specific moves meant others were to counter. There were patterns to be learned and Korean terms to be memorized. Danny and I would go over and over questions that would be on a history test. I'd drill over and over the same thing for days. The day of the test it would be gone. The therapist, the instructor, the parents and new students were, in fact, looking for the pony. Many reading this will remember the old story, one that was the basis for a television special.

The twins, one so optimistic, the other a little pessimist, who had awoke on Christmas morning to run downstairs to see what Santa had left under the tree. Their father, knowing how each viewed the world, had been determined to change their views. For the little pessimist who always anticipated the worst, he had purchased everything on the list so he could see that often good things did happen. For the little optimist who always saw the world through rose-colored glasses and who he knew would have to learn to deal with disappointments in his life, he gave only one present.

When he came down on Christmas morning, he found the little pessimist at the bottom of the stairs looking depressed. Had he not gotten him everything he asked for? Why was he so unhappy. Upon questioning, the boy responded that if he played with the bat and ball, he'd probably break a window; if he played with his bike, he'd probably strip the gears; and the results would only be that Dad would holler at him, so why bother.

We all know people like that, who make happy hour an event by not showing up, who brighten up a room by leaving it, sometimes we even marry them. But as the perplexed father listened to his son, feeling failure in his heart, he heard squeals of delight from the dining room where he had placed the lone present for his little optimist.

He scratched his head. For he knew that he had purchased, with much forethought, for his other son one present, one large box filled only with manure. How could that gift be the cause of the sounds of joy emanating from that room.

As he got up and moved to the dining room entrance, he found the little optimist down in the box and manure being slung out everywhere. It was on chairs, on the walls. Dumbfounded he stood there.

Having seen his father enter the room, the little optimist said, "Oh, Dad, isn't this great?"

And Dad could only respond, "Why would you say that? What's so great about a box of manure?"

"Oh, Dad," the boy replied. "With all this manure, there just has to be a pony in here somewhere."

The manure in our lives: parents watching our children attempt and fail; we watch them lose friends, lose their dreams, see changes in our lives, watch our dreams for them fade, many feeling life dumped a lot of that nasty stuff on our doorstep.

Determined not to let it get in our way, we, too, looked for the pony in this Martial Arts program. We had to show by our actions, that often speak louder than our words, that hope was still alive.

The class met twice a week. I sat on the sidelines. Patients who spoke before mostly the short words in passing developed a comradeship, a team approach to meeting their goal. The patterns were drilled and drilled. Danny remembered. He remembered the Korean terms; he remembered his patterns; he was once again really trying to make the uncooperative limbs work for him. This son of mine, the competitive spirit locked inside the uncooperative body, was competing again. He wanted to be a yellow belt, and he was going to be a yellow belt. Weeks went by and finally the word was go. The head injury class would test with the regular class, which was run through the recreation department in town, and Grand Master Kwang Jo Choi would be flying up from Atlanta to be one of the judges. Our class was to be tested in front of one of the leading martial arts experts in the country. It was a good thing we didn't know that then.

They were called to the front. The instructor told all in attendance that this group, all with head injuries, all having been in coma, were now to test. I was not pleased with the lengthy description of our little group, but I let it go. The test began, they watched each other; they responded to individual questions; they stood straight and remembered to say, "Yes, Sir." They each met Grand Master Choi. He wrote their names in Korean on their tobacs and complimented them on their determination. They all became yellow belts. They had achieved a goal, together they had accomplished something that was normal, and something not every uninjured person could or would do. Competitive spirit, self-esteem, a new belief system or frame of reference pushed them forward.

Danny had something to talk about at school. He couldn't play ball, but he could break boards with his hand and with his foot. He could now balance on one foot. We tested again; they received the next belt. Another test, another belt. An international martial arts magazine wanted an article. The instructor and I submitted one. I tried my hand at photography. They printed it. Our little fledgling program was now an article in an international magazine, and our little group of determined patients garnered a special place in the heart of Grand Master Choi. Never accepting loss from them, than he did the other students, he applauded their efforts and encouraged them. This fueled their determination. If he believed, they would believe. He was helping to repair their shattered belief systems in a way as parents we couldn't. We had found our pony.

Faith is a higher faculty than reason.

--Charles M. Trubac, CLU, CPCU

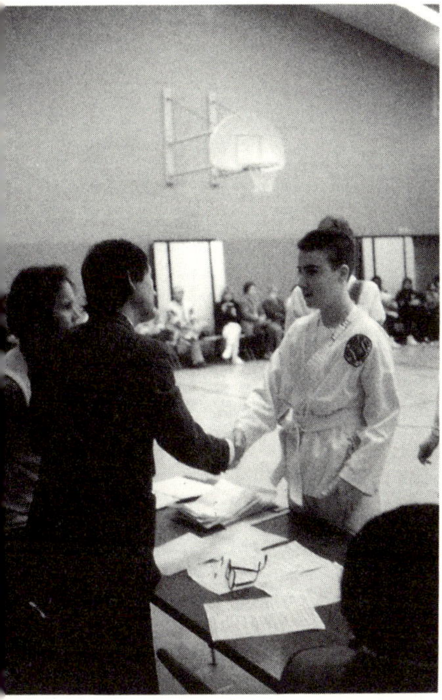

The credit belongs to the man who
is actually in the arena, whose face is
marred by dust and sweat and blood;
who strives valiantly; who errs and comes
short again and again, who knows the
great enthusiasms, the great devotions,
and spends himself in a worthy cause;
who at the best, knows the triumph
of high achievement; and who,
at the worst, if he fails, at least
fails while daring greatly, so that his
place shall never be with those cold and
timid souls who know neither victory
nor defeat.

Theodore Roosevelt

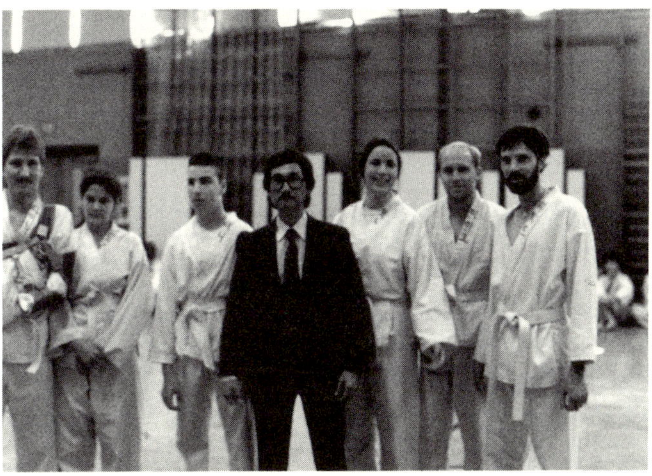

The greatest pleasure in life is doing what people say you cannot do.

--Walter Bagehot

CHAPTER 7

As Danny needed me less and less for emotional support, or to be there all the time, I found new things to fill the hours. New committees, new challenges for me personally. Anything that would keep me from thinking. The pattern I'd established when I brought Danny home from the hospital continued to plague me. I took on more. My days were now often 20 hours long, five or six days a week. When people asked me how do you get so much done, I would flippantly reply that I don't need much sleep, and I organize well. I often still scheduled appointments in my daily planner with a leeway of only ten minutes.

I put 35,000 miles a year on my car and was involved not only with Insurance Women but my church, with Cystic Fibrosis, a college insurance program, our community hospital, the head injury chapter, and anything else that came up. I was still running away. A pattern established in childhood. When it hurt, when you didn't want to deal with something, you didn't; you just ran away.

Wasn't the grass always greener somewhere else? I never stopped to think about the fact that it might have been greener because that person had stayed, nurtured and cared for it. But then I didn't want to think. It hurt too much, even when I allowed myself to do it for a few minutes.

When Danny had returned to school, we had fought for an L.D. (learning disabled) certification and won. This allowed him to receive special services and also allowed us to provide special support in the classroom. In high school, that took the form of a tutor who went to the more difficult classes, took notes and drilled Danny for tests. In high school, he also had a very special Special Ed teacher who knew how to motivate Danny and also shared Danny's unique kind of humor. In our small town, the school system worked with us, not against us, and Danny blossomed under that nurturing.

School schedules and therapy schedules filled his day. He made friends easily, but there was the normal socializing that Danny yearned for. There wasn't a special girl in his life, and the prospects didn't indicate that one was likely soon. Therapy kept us in a maintenance mode rather than one of progress. We were looking for a "pony" again. Marilyn and I spent numerous hours in meetings. We went back for another neuro-psyche evaluation, hoping for more guidance.

Danny continued to do well in his Martial Arts endeavor, and then we came to the end of his freshman year and made the transition to sophomore. His friends were beginning to take Driver's Training. Danny thought that he, too, should be allowed to take the class. I couldn't bear the idea of Danny behind the wheel of the car. What if he lost control and hit a tree? What if another driver crossed the center line? What if I had to once again sit outside an emergency room door while they fought to save his life; or worse yet, what if they didn't get the chance to try the second time. I knew in my mind and heart that if I was confronted with it again I would just die. The will to live would be sapped by the phone call. I couldn't go through all this again. I had lived the real life recovery from coma. The patient did not just wake up and walk and talk and have only some time taken from his life. Head injury more often meant weeks, months and, now I know, years to regain what one split second had taken away. I stalled. I talked to Marilyn. Danny should have a special driving instructor; we should do more reflex testing and vision checks; we shouldn't just do it through school. We'd develop a plan, go slow, but Danny would drive. Danny went along with the delays mostly because "Marilyn said".

Through all the months of recovery that we'd lived to this point, Doug's and my marriage stayed strong. We supported each other we thought. Wrong! We were both investing ourselves in Danny; we were pursuing business goals; we gave the appearance of a couple who together took on the medical community, challenged the rehab community to find new techniques, and held steadfast in support of our son and of each other. Well, we did some of that, but we were drifting apart. Did we still love each other? Yes. Did we still need each other? Maybe. Was our marriage teetering on a rocky foundation? Yes.

Doug had had enough. For some time, I had justified to him that since he bowled, hunted, and had his hobbies, that I deserved the same amount of freedom. I had finally loaded my side of the freedom scale so full that there was no balance, and Doug wanted that back and demanded I give up some of my outside involvements. How dare he ask me to give up anything! He knew how important some of those things were to me! Also, couldn't he see that the good being done in other areas outweighed the effort? Didn't making something good come out of the bad, "Danny's accident", somehow make it "not so bad"? I argued that I needed to make a difference everywhere I could. Didn't he understand my needs?

When, as a new parent, we hold that baby in our arms for the first time, we make a covenant with that child to do all in our power to give him what we never had, what we think he should have, what we think is best for him. That covenant made to that small, helpless, totally dependent baby is sometimes given to us twice in the lifetime of that same child after they sustain a head injury. Faced with starting all over again, we make a new covenant. To give to him all in our power to give. Remembering that we're the ones who must find resources, who must advocate, who must not accept what we're told only at face value. We must find the strength and courage to reach out into the unknown, where we had ventured once before. We made it then. Hadn't I brought Danny along through searching for new things, trying things that were suggested? Didn't he understand that I needed, really needed, to stay involved in all the things I was in? No, he didn't understand. I was spreading myself too thin. I was very seldom home, and when I was, I wasn't really there. I was maintaining things at the office, but even that was early morning or late night hours for the most part. The business we had both loved, the working together, once a very real and important part of our lives was now carried out in the same amount of hours, but a different time on the clock. Doug wanted the "I" that had been "we" back. He also felt that if I continued I might end up much like "The Giving Tree".

If you remember that story, there was a young man who was all alone in the world with his only possessions being the clothes on his back and a very large apple tree. The young man in the story was very unhappy and felt that the world offered him nothing. He wished for a lot of money. "If only I had money instead of this apple tree," he said aloud. Then, the apple tree spoke. "I can't give you money, but I have plenty of beautiful apples. Take them and sell them." So he picked the apples and took them to market, never saying "thank you", but the tree was happy. Sometime later, he took a wife, and still thinking life had shortchanged him, he wished aloud for a nice home. The tree spoke again. "Take my limbs for lumber. They are strong, and you can build a sturdy house." So once again, he took from the tree, never saying "thank you", built his house, and the tree was happy. Years went by and life was still not living up to his expectations. One day, sitting under the tree, whose upper limbs were not sparse, he thought of how much better life could be if he could move his family down the river, into town. The tree once again responded. "Take my trunk. You can hollow it out to make a boat so you can move farther down the river." So what remained of the beautiful tree was now cut down, save the stump. Once again there was no "thank you", but the tree was happy. The tree had given all there was to give--a classic example of unconditional love.

I had now, for months and years, been chopping away at inner reserves and resources. Doug was afraid I'd end up a stump. Looking back, the giving tree had been our marriage. I, like the young man, only wanted more. I still ran. Running to keep distance between the pain of reality and the person who was still not ready to deal with it. The tree that fueled the tree was not giving anymore.

Doug's condition for even the tenuous hold on the "stump" was to give up some of the committees, some of the activities. Be home more. And, above all, there was to be more togetherness.

I wrote resignation letters. I gave up all the least demanding positions, hoping that by doing that, I, at least, showed a willingness on my part to try. It was a ruse that didn't last long. There was more arguing.

Danny's sophomore year moved along. We had a tutor who went to classes with him, and the grades stayed up. He was seeing a psychologist to help with the struggles a young boy approaching 16 has to deal with. I'd look at Danny and remember how easy I had thought it was going to be. We were supposed to leave the hospital, Danny would wake up, we'd do therapy, and in a few months everything would be wonderful. Our own personal Dr. Kildare, Welby, or Ben Casey would be there next to us pronouncing Danny cured, with all the pomp and ceremony of a TV evangelist. It was a good thing that as we wheeled Danny from the hospital I didn't know we'd still be fighting to move forward years later.

But along with the bad news was the good news, because we had over and over again disproved the power of the myth. There was improvement after 18 months. There was improvement after three years. There was even improvement after five years. But with the good feelings, the apprehension for the future, there was within me a growing resentment. I had to give up things. Like a cut untreated by an antiseptic, it festered all through the holidays. I cooked; I entertained and shopped, spending money with a vengeance. The children and the grandchildren had the best Christmas ever at our house. Doug's wallet threatened cardiac arrest.

The new year did not appear on the horizon shining brightly and full of hope. Still angry and resentful at Doug for making me give up some of my activities, I sat at my office desk one particularly dreary January day and wrote Doug a letter. This time trying to explain my feelings, showing him in words that I had fully explored the feelings, realized the consequences, but I wanted a divorce. I could not continue as we were, and I did not believe there was any way of salvaging our marriage. While I was writing, our daughter, Denise, came in and asked what I was doing.

"Asking your father for a divorce," I replied.

She sat down in the chair across from me, tears glistening and said pleadingly, "You can't divorce Dad, you're my mother, the only one I've had all these years."

This was especially poignant to me because Denise, who was 12 when her father and I married, had, over the years, struggled through the step-parent/step-child issues. As rebellious as she could be one moment, not a more loving child could you ask for the next. There were times I hugged her and others that I restrained myself from doing her great bodily harm. Over the fifteen years or so, we had grappled with this and learned not only respect, but realized we did, in fact, love each other.

Denise and I talked for a short time, but she could not dissuade my resolve to leave Doug. Much like a small child, not given her own way, if I couldn't have mine, I'd just make everyone else miserable. If I left Doug, then I could go back to the hectic schedule and no one could stop me. Little did I know that when Denise left my office, she went immediately to her desk and typed a letter which was sent to all the other children.

The children called; they took us out to eat; they counseled with us. As strange as this role reversal was, in and of itself, it added a new richness and dimension to our lives. In this blending of families we really had become one family, and they truly were "our children". It was sad as we discovered this new closeness that we were breaking it apart.

Doug and I didn't talk. I hadn't seen an attorney, but the resolve to do so was there. We moved like people on remote control through the next two weeks. The "D" word had been said, never in all the disagreements over child rearing, money matters, family matters, business deals, purchases or philosophies had we, either of us, ever mentioned the "D" word. Now I had, and we struggled to live with it.

Our anniversary was February 6th, and Doug suggested, at the risk of being berated, that we go out to dinner. We went. Quiet table, candlelight, white wine, and the most pleasant conversation we'd had in years made for what, in my mind, was our marriage's "Swan Song". It was with emotional detachment that I saw us at the table, here on our 17th anniversary. We'd managed through all the things that tripped other people up. We'd worked together all of those years, the same goals, the same belief in what we were doing; we had had Danny, and made it through those first two years of his recovery being frustrated, tired, and worn. A couple smiling at each other over the candle, masquerading to the rest of the world, as happy. Dinner over, wine gone, the piano music about to change to something younger and noisier, we left, drove home in silence and entered the house the same way. Much like wind-up dolls, the spring that kept us animated in public had now lost its tension, and we were back to reality.

We have a rather large walk-in closet, and,as we were changing out of our party costumes, Doug took my shoulders and turned me around to face him.

Then putting his arms around me and with tears in his eyes, he said with heart-wrenching pain, "I don't want a divorce."

Upon hearing those words, the detached observer of that evening's events left for places unknown, and I found my feet planted firmly in reality. "I didn't want a divorce either." This was the man whom I'd always said I loved more than life itself. I had wanted my own way, but I knew right then it wasn't worth the price I'd have to pay to get it. Doug and I clung to each other, racked with sobs and making promises that we'd work it out. We'd loved each other for too long, been through too much, been blessed with so many things; the ship that contained all of this, as well as future promises, would not be sunk by the storms of life or the raging sea of selfish emotions. We made love that night reminiscent of the early years. Searching for pleasure but wanting to please. The storm subsiding, a full moon shown and reflected on calm waters. The love we had always whispered to each other as being "truly special" really was. We'd looked at the darkness and walked together through it back into the light. Head injury would not claim yet another victim.

Danny, although not as directly involved as our other children, had felt the strain of all this, but, through the help of a psychologist and Marilyn's support of him, the storm did no damage to the forward motion of his therapy program.

Tenth grade was good for Danny. His tutor helped with the more difficult classes, and Danny could relax a little and make friends. It always amazed me when we were in the school hallway that as other students went by Danny, they went almost out of their way to say "hi", slap hands, or some other strange thing that only teenagers do. I remember thinking, "You know you're growing old when the words coming out of your mouth are the same words you heard from your parents when you thought they were just too old to appreciate life."

Danny somehow managed to put up with me anyway. Sometimes I would look at him and wonder how such a miracle could have evolved from Doug and me. Danny went to school, then to therapy, did his homework, and seldom complained. With his dreams held in front of him, he continued the struggle with a positive attitude and a smile. What an example he set for the rest of us. He surely had been sent by the angels!

> The essence of our effort to see that every child has a chance must be to assure each an equal opportunity, not to become equal, but to become different. To realize whatever unique potential of body, mind and spirit he or she possesses.
>
> --John Fischer

I'm going to turn on the light
and we'll be two people in a room
looking at each other and wondering
why on earth we were afraid of the dark.

Gale Wilhelm

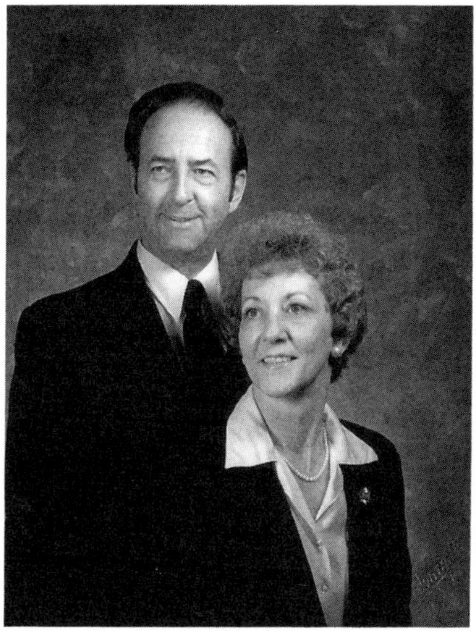

Care is Love's investment in another person
Care is love's permission for the other
to walk to the beat of a different drummer
Care is Love's gratitude for the other's unexpected gifts.
Care is Love's flexibility to go where another needs to go.
Care is Love's firmness to stay close by when the other cannot move.
Care is Love's generosity to give when the other speaks of needs.
Care is Love's presence when being there matters most.
Care is Love's power to survive the death of desire.

Lewis B. Smedes

> In the province of the mind what one believes to be true either is true or becomes true.
>
> --John Lilly

CHAPTER 8

It was time for me to really embark on an attitude adjustment. The second year of Danny's recovery process I had enrolled in a ten-week program sponsored by our community hospital, which was all about changing attitudes. I had so wanted to get a handle on mine; but even though it had served to reinforce the positive areas, I still had not mastered those which had been plaguing me for years. I kept hearing that little voice saying, "You can't change those around you, but you can change you. You can change the way you think and feel; you have control over that." Determined, I set about changing me. I adopted the attitude that I had made compromises based on saving my marriage and keeping the family unit together. I made that choice. It wasn't forced on me. When I began to look at it from that perspective, it wasn't so bad. We could build from here. I was getting more involved with the church. Doug never said anything about that. I think he was afraid to say too much about the church work. What if God were listening? I backed off in some areas but managed to find other things to build the schedule up a little. I couldn't have too much free time on my hands.

Spring came that year with all the promise that budding trees and sprouting flowers signify. Renewal, the miracle of life. How good it felt to open windows and watch the curtains billow. We had survived not only the real winter but a winter in our marriage that I hoped would never happen again. But spring brought something new. Doug began to have stomach pains. We made an appointment with the doctor.

"What kind of pain is it?" he asked.

"A pain, it hurts," was Doug's response.

"No, is it a sharp pain; a stabbing pain?" coached the doctor, trying to get Doug to be more definitive.

"It's a pain, it hurts. How do I know what kind of pain" he said grumpily.

This man, who could tell you more than you ever wanted to know about insurance, couldn't describe the pain, but was more than a little annoyed by the questions, however, had some tests run. In the meantime, the new doctor who had taken over the practice of our family physician, who had retired a few years before, was not a great believer in just medicating to medicate and took Doug off every pill he was on except those he took for narcolepsy and aspirin for some achy joints. Within three weeks, the chest pains of a few years before were back. This time it wasn't occasional. Walking out into the parking lot brought one on. We went back to the doctor. An EKG prompted him to order the standard battery.

The stress test sent us to a cardiologist who told us there was definite blockage and surgery was indicated.

In February, when Doug and I had promised to try and invest more of ourselves in our marriage, we had also begun to plan a three-week summer vacation, which was to begin the week after Danny was out of school. We had laid out a route, and, now into May, we had already told numerous people they were in our plans--some we hadn't seen for some time and one couple, our previous minister and his wife, who Doug especially wanted to see, were expecting us in June. I think Doug had wanted to see them particularly because he and David had become real friends, one of the few with whom Doug had been able to really share feelings. I know he felt he needed to talk to David, and it was with mixed emotions that I heard this salesman husband of mine negotiating with the cardiologist to at least be able to take this vacation before he had the surgery. Finally the word was yes. He could take the trip; he was to rest often, and he was not to carry heavy luggage, and monitor his activities. Doug got his way. We were going on the three-week vacation. Not only was I going to be allowed to drive more than fifty miles on this trip, which would be different (he never did like my driving), but I would get to haul all the luggage to and from the car for three weeks. This was certainly my lucky day! I also had the pleasure of wondering when the other shoe would drop. What if he had a heart attack while we were on the road, out in the middle of nowhere? What if he died out there in California? Just what if he died? I'd been willing to divorce him a few months earlier, but I knew I'd still see him, talk to him. If he died, I wouldn't have this man, who just by being next to me gave me strength. My God, what if I lost him? Danny would be devastated. His love for his father, as well as the special bond they had, fed both their spirits. Danny wouldn't go on without Doug; he'd give up; he'd settle. Oh, please, God, not now, not when we're just getting it all back together after Danny's accident that now seemed so long ago.

The day the van was finally packed and ready to go and as I hit the button to close the garage door as we were backing out of the driveway, I felt like one of the pioneer women may have felt as she rode off into the unknown. The travel was by expressway and not a wagon trail; we had air conditioning and would sleep in a bed with clean sheets and not a bed roll under the wagon; but there was no guarantee that we wouldn't be ambushed by a heart problem and waylaid along the way. We ventured forth at a pace we had never traveled before either. We stopped at various places so Doug could take a break and Danny could see some of the wonderful sights we have in these United States--Mt. Rushmore, Yellowstone, the Mississippi, Wall Drug, the Badlands; even the amber waves of grain we sing about but often fail to appreciate until you think it may be the last time. If nothing else, that trip brought us closer together and made us more appreciative of what we had and of each other.

Upon returning home, Doug was hospitalized for an angiogram. They told us that given the blockage, the test could trigger a heart attack on the table. Doug, a little dopey from medication, was wheeled away. I prayed. I couldn't lose him now. The children waited with me. Doug was through the test, and an overnight stay to watch for hemorrhaging was mandatory. He would be able to come home until the scheduled surgery date. There were four blocked arteries. The most critical was the left anterior descending. The cardiologist told us they very seldom saw that one in angiograms--it was usually in autopsies. That was the one that shut off in the cases of sudden death. And we'd gone to California?

The doctors didn't have a definite answer as to what had caused this blockage. There had been no high blood pressure, cholesterol was 130 with all the right values for triglycerides and lipids. Doug had never been a heavy smoker, but stress could also cause this and the pressure from chasing the carrots held out by the company for the contests, recognition, plaques, not to mention competitiveness had long driven Doug. At one time, he had been the top agent in Michigan. He'd work as hard for a set of coffee cups or an umbrella as he would for a trip. It wasn't so much the prize that was offered, it was achieving the goal over the other agents.

There's no way to measure the toll Danny's accident had taken on Doug's health, but we had gotten medical attention in time and only the operation loomed before us.

I requested more psychological counseling for Danny, so we could start preparing him mentally for his father's surgery. He also needed to at least be aware that something could happen on the table, or Dad might be different after this. I had seen open heart surgery on TV, and I kept thinking, "What if they can't jump start the heart after they do all the patching?"

The day of the surgery once again the children rallied. The girls and I sat and worried. Our three macho sons sat there talking and acting smug in their private knowledge that Dad would be just fine. Several hours later the doctor came in to tell us it had all gone well. Doug was in recovery and would be put in the Cardiac Intensive Care unit soon, and we could see him. The girls and I hugged each other and shared tears of relief and thankfulness. Our sons smiled and said, "See, we told you it'd be okay. Dad's tough."

Doug didn't look tough as I went into the Intensive Care Unit to kiss him goodbye and go home to make phone calls all over the country to let people know he was through it. The doctor said he should be out for another 10 or 12 hours so not to plan on being back too early in the morning. I thought he knew what he was talking about; so after the calls were made, I set my alarm for seven hours later and fell into bed to sleep the sleep that only exhaustion brings.

Morning came too soon for my body, but I needed to see that Doug was okay and talk to him. So I got ready, letting those staying at the house with me know I was on my way to the hospital. My heels clicked out their usual "I'm in a hurry" song down the hospital corridors. I hit the automatic door button for the unit and headed for Doug's bed, figuring I still had time before he was taken off the respirator and fully awake. Wrong again. He was wide awake, looking at me as I walked toward the head of the bed.

"Where the hell have you been?" he growled. "I've been awake for two hours. They took me off that thing, and you weren't here."

I tried to explain that according to the doctor last night he shouldn't be awake and talking yet. I was sorry; I had believed them. What did he want me to do? Get him a basin, he was sick. I was so glad he'd waited until I got there so he could share that with me. (That was always the worst part of mothering for me.) But you do learn, and I held the pan, wiped his face, and hoped I was now off the hook.

We had been told before the surgery that Doug would probably spend most of the day in that unit. But now they were changing the plans. He was doing so well, he was going to a room as soon as they got a bed ready. Two hours and he was all set up with tubes and monitors in a regular room, and all the kids were there.

Dad was feeling pretty chipper, and he moved around in the bed. Then he noticed that if he moved just right, it showed on the monitor; and if he held his breath, he could get a straight line. The straight line set off an alarm, and the nurse came running. Danny and Doug encouraged their Dad, and Dad entertained for several hours. Finally the nurses came in and turned his monitor so he couldn't play games, and told him no visitors the next day. Period. Doug was doing fine; it was going to be okay. We'd have mending time, but it was going to be okay.

We'd just gotten our second miracle. The first one sat and laughed with the man now in the hospital bed. A role reversal. Thank you God. They were both talking this time. We'd gotten to the doctor in time; he'd taken Doug off the Inderol that had effectively been masking the problem. A few more months, and he could have just fallen over at the dinner table, or at the office, and we'd never known. This was the second time had the sequence of events been different, death might have been the victor. (The first being Danny's injury--doctors at the scene giving mouth-to-mouth resuscitation until the paramedics arrived, the availability of a trauma center so close--reinforced my belief in miracles, even though I still prayed for Danny's full recovery.) Bad things may, in fact, happen to good people; but with faith, family, friends and all the things available within our community, we are often better for the experience. I was better for mine. I would have traded everything we owned, or hoped to own, our health, anything, to put things right for Danny. But not then, not even now would I change one of the things for me.

Now, I had two in rehab and soon would have one more. Doug's mother, in her eighties, was still maintaining her independence, living alone in a remodeled cottage located on an island on a lake about a half hour away. The property had once been part of Doug's grandfather's farm, had passed down through the generations and we looked forward to it becoming our retirement home one day. Given mom's age, we were not happy with her being alone; but we also felt that her pressing need for independence was what kept her alive. We had a special system installed so that all she had to do was push a button and a call was made to the local hospital. They, in turn, called a neighbor who would check on her. This time, though, it was grandma who called. She was in pain and needed help. I left at once and took her to the Emergency Room. Diagnosis, twisted bowel, surgery was required, and she would be admitted immediately. I filled out forms, got her settled, went home and checked on Doug, made arrangements for Danny, and cleared things at the office. I didn't ask God why on this one. Grandma was old. We had known for years, since Doug was an only child, that her care would fall to us, and that was okay. The tiny gray-haired lady, growing more stooped every year, had never defined our relationship in in-law terms. I was never just Doug's wife or second wife; I was always her daughter. Although I didn't have a lot of patience with the repetition or the loss of hearing, I had grown to love her, and she had her own special place in my heart. Super-woman was on the job. All would be okay. Doug went to visit her in the hospital. When she was able to be discharged, we once again set up a bedroom/sitting room in the living room, and grandma joined Doug in recuperating.

They healed together. As Doug was ready to drive and go back to work, we moved grandma home with a list of instructions and new items--a cart to push things on so she didn't have to carry, a cane to move around with during the day, and a walker to use at night. We wouldn't take away her independence if she did these little things.

Doug was to continue with the heart rehab program, but he could now drive and be back to work. We made a special point to work. We made a special point to send letters out to all our clients and thank them for, once again, calling and caring for our family through a crisis. We saved all the cards and phone slips to be put in a scrapbook later. How fortunate we felt, once again, to be in a business where caring could play such an integral part. Super-woman was, for the most part, out of a job. Did that seem reasonable? For a few days, maybe even a few weeks, I think I was too tired, worn down again, to care. But energy came back and this, Danny's junior year in high school, found us faced with more changes in Danny's life.

Danny's therapy program, which had initially been a small community-based program through Saline Hospital, was moving to the big city, to become part of a national firm. Danny would continue with the regular school classes; he would have a tutor at least 4 hours of that day, and then would have a co-op job and the continued therapy. Now much taller than I and becoming more assertive, he played an active role in his rehab. The Martial Arts class continued. He was passing each test, each with a belt of a different color, and was having a social life of sorts.

Doug and I had addressed our personal problems with more than a bandaid this time. All was looking much better than it had for years. We had been brought up short by the heart surgery. We tried to grasp that new perspective. The one that addresses "Life is just too short to": keep pushing so hard at work, to feel like you always had to be busy at home, to put any number of things before family. I've never been a salesman, never really wanted to be, but I sold this concept hard, just short of demanding it. We'd been a team for almost twenty years; I couldn't bear to contemplate life without Doug in it. Danny needed his father there to cheer him on, to validate his often small victories as he worked his way along the long road to recovery. We began to share in Danny's rehab, really share for the first time. There were team meetings and insurance company meetings, and we faced them together. It felt so good to not be doing it alone. I wondered why I had thought I had to take it on by myself for so long. Although I now shared this with Doug, I had become active with the Insurance Women again, was working in several areas of our church, and also quite actively involved at a local and state level with the Michigan Head Injury Alliance.

Through Danny's marketing class, he was part of a group of students who ran the school store. I'd drop him off at 7:30 in the morning and go to the office. The free time with no phone gave me time to organize my day, which was about 18 hours long. Super-woman was re-emerging, and this time with a vengeance. There was so much to do, and so little time. My favorite saying became "Who needs sleep?" I'll sleep for a long time some day. I don't need it now, and I didn't feel like I did. With Danny's life now seemingly running more smoothly, his needing me less and less for monitoring but still for transportation and caregiving, there was once again an increase in free time. There were problems in our church and problems in Insurance Women I thought I could challenge and challenge I did. I became part of the "Pulpit Committee" to search for a new pastor, and I started writing letters addressing the issues with Insurance Women, sometimes sending out four or five hundred copies across the country. This allowed me to do a couple of things: keep busy, fill up the hours, but feel like I was giving back to this group of women who had cared for me, not only as a professional but as a person, for years. My new buzz word became "sheep". (Sheep, not very bright animals, while in a flock will often follow blindly, not thinking for themselves and would continue off the edge of a cliff if it weren't for the shepherd.) I felt as members of this organization, we were behaving the same way, and I set about to make a difference. Hadn't I, with dogged determination, made a difference in Danny? Had I not, through that same determination, passed classes, developed new skills, taken care of my family, ran my home, managed the office? There she was. Super-woman was back on the job.

The letters rolled out; letters came in. Doug, for a change, was supportive of the flurry of activity in which I found myself. I had never felt better. I often said to people, if I had a choice to be any age, I'd be exactly here. Secure in self and my marriage. Job going well--the 40's were great years. Besides, there was only one child still in the nest, Danny, and he would someday be on his own, with the dogs right behind. It just didn't get any better than this. I had a cause to fight for, one I truly believed in, a commitment to these women who had cared for me over the years. My body ran on super-charge.

If I had a formula for bypassing trouble, I would not pass it round. Trouble creates a capacity to handle it.

I don't embrace trouble; that's as bad as treating it as an enemy.

But I do say meet it as a friend, for you'll see a lot of it and had better be on speaking terms with it.

--Oliver Wendell Holmes

> The last of the human freedoms to choose one's attitude in any given set of circumstances, to choose one's own way.
>
> --Victor Frank

CHAPTER 9

Things did look good for Danny. He still had a crazy gait pattern that no one could seem to correct. His left arm still gave him problems but successes in the school store made his eyes sparkle. He knew he wanted to be a business man, take business classes in college, and get married some day. Therapy was decreasing; Danny's days approached normalcy. He had a part-time job in a men's clothing store and, being blessed with an inner confidence and strong verbal skills, he got along well. All this led me to hope, more than I had ever dared before, that it really would be okay for Danny. It really would be okay.

Rehab team meeting--the physical therapist said Danny didn't need therapy; the Choi Kwang Do class was enough. The occupational therapist did not believe any more could be done in therapy for his hand. Other than job skills, help with school, social skills, Danny could be sent out in the community, according to the doctor. Only limited therapy was required, besides one hour of psyche time per week, to give Danny a vent for frustration other than his family. I sat in that meeting numb. Once again, the medical profession had torn our comfortable walls down from around us. We were going to be not cut off from the professional contact daily, but it would be limited. Danny would no longer do Choi Kwang Do at therapy time; he would take it through the Community Ed program. He would continue his job, and we would still strive for cognitive improvement. But the physical, well, it might get better; but there were not going to be any efforts in therapy. I not only was scared at losing this comfortable, safe haven, I felt alone, betrayed by the medical community. Danny wasn't 100%; they hadn't made him completely better. How could the doctor and therapist sit there and recommend no more therapy?

Sometimes the family, if they've been lucky, will have a physical medicine rehabilitation physician as well as therapists who will tell you, "I, or we, have taken the patient one step further, but you need to look at alternatives, and even offer to aid in the search for that next step." Conventional therapy does not always reign supreme in the unconventional situations survivors of TBI or the families find themselves. Unconventional methods, like the bubble gum wrapped in gauze that kicked in Danny's ability to chew, are being tried every day by physicians, nurses and therapists all over the country as this, the "Silent Epidemic", creeps up on thousands of families every year in this country. Those in the rehab business share their knowledge through conventions, publications, and continuing education vehicles. "If it can't hurt, it's worth a try" had always been our philosophy. We had tried surgery, alcohol blocks, hypnosis, biofeedback, exercise, range of motion by a computerized unit, Choi Kwang Do, Special Ed, tutors, and invested ourselves. Danny still walked with a strange gait, his left arm was only functional as an aide to the right arm, not independent. There were still some unresolved memory problems, and learning road blocks. "Where, dear Lord, do we go from here?" I asked that evening, as I sank into a fitful sleep.

The next morning, as I sat at my desk, I could see the framed copy of "Footprints", given to me by an old friend several years before. I knew I needed carrying for awhile. So many weeks, months, years. We certainly had made a great deal of progress. My 5'11" cauliflower was about to enter his senior year in high school; he would graduate with the same young people he'd started kindergarten with. He was a warm, caring, unselfish young man. He had a strong sense of self and never had allowed himself to believe there was anything he couldn't do, if he wanted to bad enough. But I knew that belief systems change when confronted day after day with road blocks. Also, we couldn't let Danny settle, nor get used to doing nothing. Early in Danny's therapy/recovery, I'd heard the story about the "Self-fulfilling Prophesy". This was not going to be the case if there were any alternatives. Once again, at my side, was my friend, the "miracle lady", Marilyn, assuring me that there were some options in physical as well as occupational therapy and that she was, along with two others, opening a new program. We'd find a way.

Marilyn and I had become friends through these years from 1982 to 1989. We had shared professional as well as personal successes and tragedies. When Danny became her patient, her son was the same age. A bond grew between them that years or miles will never destroy. I used to tease Doug and say that if anything ever happened to me that Danny would put pressure on him to marry Marilyn so he could have the two people he loved most in all the world around him all the time. Doug would laugh, but I was sure that would be the case if anything ever did happen to this person I was coming to believe could handle anything. What could possibly happen to me? I didn't have time to be sick and had too much to do yet to even consider dying. The day Danny was born, I made a commitment to love and care for him until his own growth process drew him away from me. I renewed that commitment when I took him home from the hospital in a coma, as well as every road block we'd had during his recovery to date. Keeping that commitment each time helped to keep hope alive in me, and I hoped I could also do that for Doug and Danny by pursuing other avenues.

Danny, now seventeen, began to want some control of his own. He also wanted to have a say in his activities. As a Senior, he would help manage the school store; so we were on the road at 7:15 every school day. He was determined that he would drive, and I should stop treating him like a baby. I promised to push the driving with a special instructor, not the regular school program. He also let me know that he was going out for the football team. Football, driving, another injury? Well, that would surely push me over the edge.

Just what I needed, to start over again, if I were lucky, that was, lucky enough to have him survive a second time. I didn't want to say yes, but I couldn't say no to this son of mine who kept "looking for that pony" and, through his positive attitude, drew others along with him.

> My mother had a great deal of trouble with me, but I think that she enjoyed it.
>
> --Mark Twain

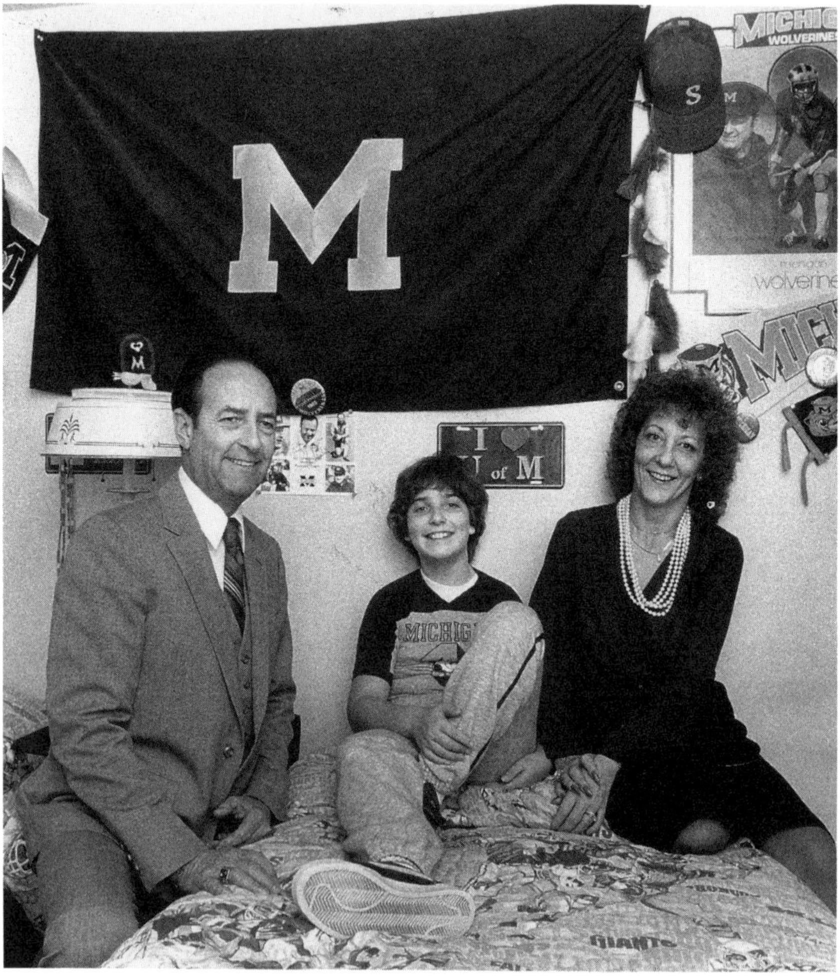

A person who is severely impaired never knows his hidden source of strength until he is treated like a normal human being and encouraged to shape his own life.

--Helen Keller

It is common sense to take a method and try it. If it fails audit it and try another. But above all try something.

--Franklin D. Roosevelt

CHAPTER 10

"I'm on the team, Mom," were words that greeted me one afternoon. Coach won't let me play, but he says I can be a team manager and help the guys with equipment and be with the team. "It will be great, Mom, just being with the guys. It's going to be great, Mom, and I can get my Varsity letter and a jacket. You'll have to get me to practices, Mom. You're coming to watch the team play; aren't you, Mom?" Danny had certainly started to make his senior year memorable.

That spring I had been elected Regional Vice President for the Insurance Women's organization. This meant from June of 1989 to June of 1990, I would work with and travel in four states for the local associations. October, the height of football season, I would be gone every weekend, but I promised that Dad would be there and when I could, I would. My favorite way to watch football had always been via television, not out in the cold. I hoped it wouldn't dampen Danny's spirits when I wasn't there. It didn't.

The long hours on his feet, with the left foot at an odd angle, as well as carrying heavy equipment bags, caused Danny pain. He would come home at night angry and hurting, wanting to either break the ankle or just cut it off. We wrapped the foot in an ace bandage and began freezing water in Dixie cups, as we had a long time ago to ice aching muscles. Danny alternated ice and heat on the now raging ankle, but he was there at every practice, every game, encouraging the players to do their best, cheering them on, and slapping high fives with the guys. He couldn't be on the team, but he could be with the guys. For Danny, it was worth the pain he endured.

I traveled and kept up my usual schedule. Most nights Danny got a ride home from practice. He was fairly independent now, so I only needed to be around for the essentials--meals and laundry and occasional help with dressing. After all, he was a senior.

"I'm a jock, Mom. Well, I'm not playing, but I'm part of the team. The guys are great, Mom. You know what the coach said, Mom? I help keep 'em going, Mom."

Danny had not been this vocal or animated in years. This was so good for Danny; he was doing more normal things. The Martial Arts class through the City schools was also going well. Danny was being accepted as one of the Club, his personality overcoming what he lacked in physical ability. Danny was doing well in spite of all of his mother's fears. He was driving with an instructor twice a week. This was surely starting out to be a great year for Danny, and his success and my now even-busier schedule made this a banner year for me, also. For the first time, there was almost no pain in my heart when I looked at Danny and mourned his losses. He didn't appear to be mourning anymore, and it was apparent that it was time for me to give it up.

Yes, it was apparent I should not feel bad because Danny, who had been born with natural athletic ability--had led all the little leagues in home runs for the season the year before his accident, had dreamed of being quarterback for the U of M, had slept with footballs or ball gloves under walls draped with Michigan maize and blue objects--would probably never realize the dream; he was seizing life and teaching his mother some of the most basic facts of life therein; life is not always fair; and that when life gave Danny a real lemon, he chose to make lemonade now that he was old enough to have some say; and since he was pouring, I should just drink. I drank; life was good, not always fair, but certainly good.

Tonight was the sports banquet. All the team members were to be recognized and awards and letters were to be presented. Marilyn and I sat side by side in the auditorium, waiting to see the child I gave to the world through birth and the child she gave back to the world through patience, training, and love, walk across the stage. The coach called Danny's name, and he walked up to get his letter, one foot right in front of the other. He was really concentrating to make that happen. How proud we were as we listened to praise for his positive attitude, untiring efforts, and support for the team. My cauliflower left the stage with a varsity letter for football. I didn't know then it was going to cost me three hundred dollars for the jacket it was to be attached to.

Those presentations over, as well as ones given by the team members, the team captain came to the podium. There was to be a special presentation that evening. The local cable station and sporting goods store had gone together and designed a tee shirt that was to be given to the player of the week so he could wear it during the following week and be recognized for his accomplishment, as well as bask in warmth that only comes when you are chosen for recognition by your peers. There were only enough shirts for each week of football, and there were to be no others made. But there was one in the hand of the team captain that night and, through eyes clouded by tears, he called the last member to be recognized by the team that year, Danny Hoppe. As they embraced, two senior boys, soon to be men of the world, in the center of the auditorium stage, Mom lef the auditorium with a lump in her throat so big she thought it would burst. It was a truly special evening. All the pain Danny had endured for the past weeks in his arm and ankle and in that deep down part of us no one sees, as he watched his buddies play a game he never would play but cheered them on, this had not gone unrecognized by the team of special young men who had learned to look beyond outside appearance or sports ability and see what makes us all so uniquely us.

They had in that moment made it worth it all for Danny and for me. I needed air.

As tears rolled down my cheeks in the cool fall air, I lifted my eyes and once again asked God, "Why? Hadn't we worked hard enough, long enough? Why can't you just touch his head and make it better? Why? Why? Why?" As I was railing internally, my long-time friend and Danny's guide through the rehab maze, Marilyn, took my arm. The silence was shattered as I shouted at God about how unfair it was that all these things had to happen to Danny and could he not have spared Danny that pain. "Why? Why? Why?" As tears blurred both our visions, her calm voice, the one that quieted the unreasonable patient, brought me back to the reality of the moment and I quieted down. If Danny never played ball, at least we had Danny, so special in his own way, I should let it go. If Danny could begin to, so should I. Emotions were quickly brought under control, given guidance, and tucked back away in the box that I felt had been established and kept solely for all those painful feelings. The name on the outside read "Danny". When we got home, we starting putting the football memorabilia aside to make yet another scrapbook to add to the collection.

The Choi Kwang Do classes continued. Danny was now three tests away from black belt. He was doing very well in the regular classes, and the comradeship that the patients had had was now being replaced by even more of the same, under normal conditions. This was a good move. Danny blossomed under the new friendships and acceptance.

There were martial arts students who were also in Danny's high school, and it broadened that base for Danny, as well. The stretches and exercises required before class helped to keep Danny limber, helped to further stretch the very tight hamstrings. Maybe Danny had really needed this break from the endless rounds of therapy to just be a kid.

We had settled into another very comfortable routine, and I kept my daily planner still full within 15 minute intervals. Doug and I had established new ground rules. Even though we each had many projects of our own, Danny was a central focus. The ships who passed back and forth during the 24-hour nights did stop occasionally to see a movie or have dinner before going on our respective ways.

During the football season, there were five weeks that I never really unpacked my suitcase. I'd take dirty clothes out and leave everything else, where I used it as needed. I came home on Sunday and would leave the next Thursday. Doug endured and worked around my schedule. It ended during the holidays, and I decorated the house and planned parties. I also did, once again, one of my favorite Christmas things, spend money.

The man who had hired Doug as an agent had recently passed away, and, as I rang up charge slips, I remembered what he had told me when Doug and I married. "Go out and buy anything you want; Doug can sell enough to pay for it." I'm sure if I had been a manager who received an override off agents' sales or the ones that I knew were able to, I may have used that ploy, also. It certainly had worked for him at our house. I knew how to do it well and became even better at it as I justified some purchases for Danny. I also used the "the way I dress indicates how successful you are" and "I'm only doing it for you" ploy. It took me 17 years to get him to realize I needed a mink coat. It was my Christmas present that year, and I wrote checks every month to pay for it for many months after, but I had the long-awaited mink.

The holidays over, the new year dawned with great promise. Danny was doing well in school with the help of a tutor and would graduate right on schedule with his class. We were seeing positive changes in the cognitive area as he was exposed to more things out in the real world. He was driving with a special instructor on a regular basis, and the reports were encouraging. Danny would probably be a safe driver, so all I had to worry about were the hundred thousand or so uninsured and/or unlicensed drivers with tickets, accidents, or a history of drunk driving out on the road on any given day who might run into him. No problem! I could push that in various 10-minute intervals in my daily planner.

When Danny was born, he became the whole family's baby. He united all our children and bound us all together into the ever growing family, which now claimed nine grandchildren. If we kept growing, Doug would have to keep working just to rent a hall for the holidays and other family events. His suggestion of hooks on the wall for each of the kids was just out of the question.

I picked Danny up from school one day as winter was reluctantly making its exit. "I'm going to try out for the baseball team, Mom. I have to be at school at six in the morning" was coming out of Danny's mouth as he seated himself and hooked up the seat belt.

"You're what?" was my response. I couldn't believe my ears. Why would Danny put himself through this? I knew his off kilter, loping run would not serve him well; and his left arm still did not respond even when we got the glove on over uncooperative fingers, like the coach would want him anywhere in the outfield. Why did he want to put himself through this? As I look back now, it might have been more honest if I'd said, "Why me?" also. I didn't think I could bear to read disappointment on his face one more time. But I had also learned a real respect for the "determination to try" in this son of mine as I'd watched him learn to walk, to ride a bike again, to pitch to his Dad. If he failed, it would never be because he didn't try and try 150%. Many times the student teaches the teacher, and this was just another lesson for Mom.

When Danny was still involved with the local hospital head injury program, Marilyn and I had arranged, through a motivational professional who worked with high school sports teams, to put together a series of weekly sessions for the head injury patients. Their theme after three or four weeks became "You gotta want it <u>and</u> you gotta want it bad"--they said it; they meant it, and we saw renewed interest in therapy. Danny wanted it, and he wanted it bad. Keep your mouth shut, Mom, just drive. He's old enough to have some choices of his own.

We got Danny to the early morning practices, and he stayed after his last class and waited for the afternoon practice. We'd put the remaining therapies on hold for ball season, or at least while Danny tried out for the team. The ankle was raging once again, but Danny wouldn't give up. Cuts were made; the team was chosen.

"Coach said he'd like to let me play, Mom, but he was just afraid I'd get hurt again. But it's okay, Mom, he says I can be an assistant and still be part of the team. I'll be with the guys, Mom."

My heart broke for Danny, a lump filled my throat again and does now as I write this. No one ever told me life was fair. I didn't expect it to be; but didn't this boy, my son who kept trying, kept his dream alive, deserve to have one of the medical breakthroughs that occur around the world every day be the one that would help him. God and I would talk again that afternoon. Danny got on with the business of living while I wallowed for two or three days in the blues for him. My son was teaching me over and over that failure wasn't not meeting your goal, but failure was not trying. He had to try, and he accepted what he got, much more gracefully than I did. Being on the baseball team as an assistant at least got Danny a uniform that he wore proudly, a special shirt he was to wear on game days and a sweatshirt. He wore them proudly and kept up his now very busy schedule.

Doug and I worked out a driving schedule for ball, therapy, and school, which we shared because I was on the road as much that spring as I had been the previous fall with Insurance Women. I had even determined that since Danny would be through school in June, I would run for a position on the National

Board and put a campaign into motion, started making graduation plans for Danny, and went shopping for a pickup truck. Didn't take very long to find some to look at. Danny's driving instructor had agreed with us that a small pickup, where Danny would be limited to one passenger to eliminate distraction and a small engine to eliminate speed, was a pretty good bet for this young man who now was the proud holder of a driver's permit which allowed him to drive with a licensed driver. We felt it would serve two purposes if we bought a vehicle now. One, his Dad could ride with him as he drove it; and by the time he had the long-awaited license, he'd be used to the vehicle; and we could feel better having him on the road alone when the time came. Truck found, deal made, and papers signed, Danny became the proud owner of a used Chevy S10 with a pretty good body and new tires. He couldn't drive alone yet, but all his buddies knew he had a truck.

No one can know the potential of a life that is
committed to win;
With courage . . . the challenge it faces to achieve
great success in the end!

So, explore the dimensions of greatness, and believe
that the world can be won;
By a mind that is fully committed, knowing the task
can be done!

Your world has no place for the skeptic, no room for
the doubter to stand;
To weaken your firm resolution, that you can excel in
this land!

We must have vision to see our potential, and faith to
believe what we see;
Then courage to act with conviction, to become what
God meant us to be!

So possess the strength and the courage, to conquer
whatever you choose;
It's the person who never gets started, that is destined
forever to lose!

--Dr. Heartsill Wilson

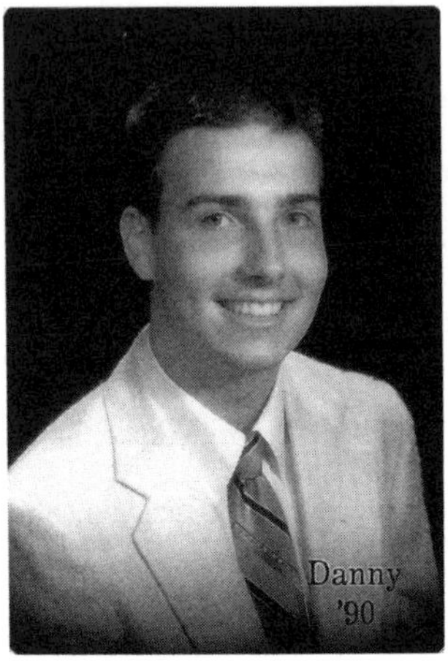

WINNER V S LOSER

The winner is always part of the answer
the loser is always part of the problem.
The winner always has a program
the loser always has an excuse.
The winner says "Let me do it for you".
The loser say s "That's not my job".
The winner sees an answer for
every problem
The loser see s a problem for every answer.
The winner sees a green near every
sandtrap.
The loser sees two or three sand
traps near every green.
The winner says "It may be difficult
but its possible."
The loser says "It may be possible
but it will be difficult."

He Helps Breathe Life into Program

Danny Hoppe, a patient in the Saline Community Hospital Head Trauma Program, took first place in the Youth Division during the annual "Bowl-for-Breath" bowl-a-thon, sponsored by the Washtenaw County Chapter of the Cystic Fibrosis Foundation.

Hoppe, a three-year veteran of the CF annual drive, previously collected pledges while his father did the bowling. This year, Hoppe bowled for the first time and and won a color television for his efforts. He donated the set to the Saline Chapter of the Michigan Head Injury Alliance April 20. Hoppe stated that, since he already had a set, he thought it would be nice for the families in the program to have a way to view informational videotapes.

Hoppe has been in the program for five years and has made a great progress since the first time when he indicated he was collecting the money for CF for "kids who have less chance than I do," according to a spokesman for the Saline Chapter of the Michigan Head Injury Alliance.

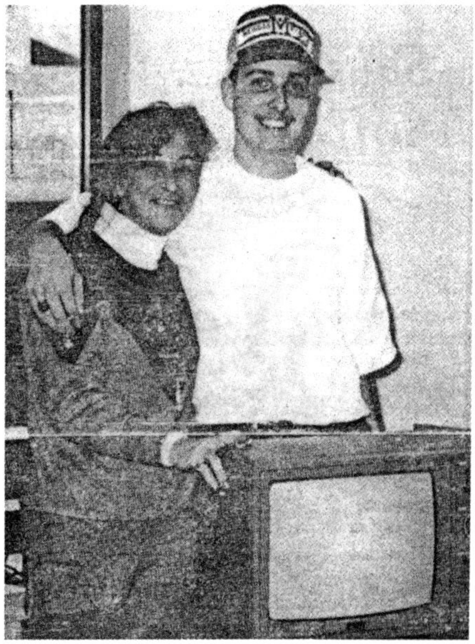

I'd rather see a sermon than hear one anyday.
I'd rather one should walk with me than merely point the way.
Because the eye is a better pupil and more willing than the ear,
Fine counsel is confusing but your examples always clear.
And the best of all the preachers, are the men that live their creed,
for to see good put into action, that's what everybody needs.
And I can soon learn how you do it, if you'll show me how it's done.
I can watch your hands in action, but your words too fast can run.
And those lectures you deliver, may be very wise and true,
but I'd rather get my lesson by observing what you do.
For I could misunderstand you, and that great advice you give,
but there's no misunderstanding, how you act, and how you live.

Edgar Guest

> To laugh often and much; to win the respect of intelligent people and the affection of children; to earn the appreciation of honest critics and endure the betrayal of false friends; to appreciate beauty; to find the best in others; to leave the world a bit better whether by a healthy child, a garden patch, or a redeemed social condition; to know even one life has breathed easier because you have lived. This is to have succeeded.
>
> --Ralph Waldo Emerson

CHAPTER 11

For years, Danny had taken part in my work with the local Cystic Fibrosis Foundation. He'd taken special Christmas cards around the neighborhood to sell before his accident and felt good about the part he'd played in raising funds for research. When fund raising changed from Christmas cards to my Insurance Women's Association doing a fashion show, he'd missed helping with the cards. That spring after his accident, he found a new way to help. Every spring there was a Bowl for Breath. Danny decided on his own that he could collect the pledges, and his Dad could bowl for him since he was still functioning most of the time in a wheelchair. He'd rehearsed his plea for pledges over and over again, now for the seventh year. Even with baseball, he went out to collect the pages of pledges, more committed than ever this year. Danny, early on, even when his steps were halting, wanted to help children he felt were less fortunate than himself. Collecting pledges and convincing Dad to bowl and then going back to collect the money was one thing Danny could do, and he did it with the zeal that only those who not only make, but understand the meaning of commitment know.

I heard a speaker years ago tell a story about commitment, or lack of it. There was once a businessman who cared only about himself, and,to aid his ego, he also went after the big deals, the big games in life. He had never been a hunter, but,when this man did decide he would like to do that, he only wanted to hunt the big game. Having decided to go bear hunting, he contracted with a preserve to do just that. There would be no small game for this hunter; he only wanted once again to capture a big prize, much the same as he did in business. Once out in the woods, the inexperienced hunter became the hunted as a big grizzly spotted him, before he spotted the bear. Despite dropping everything and running as fast as he could, when the dust settled, the bear was planted firmly on the hunter's chest with his paw about to strike the hunter's throat. This hunter, who was so eager to close big deals, who never bothered to make any commitments and never one to his Maker, whom he thought he might be meeting soon, decided if he ever were going to make a commitment, he'd better do it now. Closing his eyes tight, he said, "Dear Lord, please, make this bear a Christian!" As he opened his eyes to see if, by chance, a miracle had occurred, there sat the grizzly, paws now together, toes pointing upward, while saying, "Thank you, Lord, for this meal I'm about to receive."

Danny seemed to know about this instinctively as he went about his annual appeal for pledges. For two years, Dad bowled. The third year Danny bowled, and that year collected enough money to place in the prizes. He won an Atari system, and since, he had one, he donated it to the therapy program. His third year of bowling, the prize was a color TV set. Since he also had one of those, he donated it to the Saline Chapter of the Michigan Head Injury Alliance to use to view information videos. His commitment, his caring, taught many of us. Danny worked to get the prizes, not for the prize which he so often gave away, but just for the sake of winning it. The competitive spirit within his uncooperative body just wouldn't die.

That spring, even though he had made the ball team, he collected his pledges. Although there were several hundred dollars collected, he hadn't garnered first prize but second was okay. He told me missing first did not matter because that senior year had given him first-hand knowledge of this disease that kills children. One of his classmates, a lovely young lady, became another of its victims, and Danny felt good because every dollar helped.

Danny was well-liked once again by his teammates, and several of them went to the coach to try and get him to put Danny into a real game, if only for an inning. Danny made friends easily but kept them, I believe, because he knew how to be a friend, and the feelings ran full circle.

I was out of town, in Ohio again, for an association function--this time in recognition of National Insurance Women's Week and called home to check on my two favorite fellows. Danny answered the phone. When I asked how the game had gone, Danny could hardly contain himself.

"Coach put me in the game, Mom. I got to play. I got to play in a game, Mom."

I couldn't believe what I was hearing. The coach had said Danny didn't make the lineup. What was going on? Doug assured me that Danny, suited up, glove on, had been put in at the end of the game as an outfielder. He had indeed been in the game. What we found out much later was the coach, whom we had known for years, a wonderfully caring man, had in fact put Danny's name on the roster and kept it there just in case there was ever an opportunity where he could put Danny on the field in a safe situation. Danny had never given up, and he had, indeed, been on the field with his buddies; and they celebrated with him after the game. I hung up the phone that night so thankful for even that little bit of recognition for Danny. I thought it was little; he thought it was worth it all. He still had some more teaching to do.

The "All Sports" spring banquet was the highlight for May. All the teams were recognized, and the baseball team had their special spot. I vowed that I would not leave this time to go outside and question God. If Danny wasn't, how dare I. When coach finished his presentations to the "most valuable player" and the other categories, he had one more presentation. In his hand he held a dirty baseball and in his eyes was a glisten that hinted of tears. This coach, who had always taught sportsmanship and fair play along with the skills necessary to achieve a win, had also taught our sons caring and friendship. He said, "The next player not only supported the team, but taught them lessons in living life as well".

He then called Danny's name. With a smile that brightened the room Danny walked to the coach, hugged him and proudly accepted his award. This was the ball Danny had chased in his one inning played in that season which was recovered by his teammates and put away just for Danny. This was his game ball, which will probably always have a place of honor in any home Danny ever has for it represents much more than a ball hit to the outfield; it represents perseverance, determination, and an unwillingness to give up a dream. It also represents the importance of a good coach in teaching sportsmanship, as well as friendship and fellowship, to young men who have grown into caring individuals and who know how to use what they're taught.

It had only been three weeks or so before, that my elected and also unpaid, duties as a Regional Vice President for the Insurance Women took me to Kentucky, where I presided over a Regional Conference where my successor would be elected. As I have always believed that if you have good people, you stay out of their way and let them do their job, I tried to stay out of the way of the Insurance Women of Louisville as much as possible as they planned and put together the 1990 Conference. I had asked only for the opportunity to make one special presentation and to make an introduction at the closing banquet. As the Conference approached, I was knee deep in an estate sale as Doug's mother, now requiring 24-hour care, had been placed in a home and could no longer live with us, and we needed to liquidate assets to provide for her. (That experience in and of itself would provide book material.) I was sending out the usual campaign propaganda that those people who like to work harder for no money than they do to earn a living traditionally were required to send out, and I had a graduation coming up that Danny had every intention of making a big, as well as costly, event. We were also working with a local body shop to armorize (by way of roll bars, brush bars and heavy-duty bumpers) Danny's little red truck. Since Sherman tanks weren't allowed on state highways, we had decided to design our own.

Danny and Doug arrived in Louisville the morning of the banquet and would spend the night to drive home early the next day and let me wrap things up at my own speed. So intent on protocol and following the mandatory script book, I had forgotten to make myself notes for the introduction. As I stood waiting to be placed in position for the head table lineup, I made notes on a napkin.

There were to be three very important people at the banquet that night: One, the CEO of the insurance company who had been supportive of women in the industry for years, and my mentor, as I'd worked with the Association and the industry in the State of Michigan. Two, my husband of almost 20 years, who early on had given me problems with my involvement but had always encouraged personal growth and through all these years of Danny's recovery, even when I had been at my most unreasonable stages, continued to love me unconditionally and was always proud of what I did accomplish. The most important person in that room that night was the last to be introduced. As I scribbled on the napkin earlier, the only thing that kept coming to mind was the words of a song from the movie, "Beaches": "Did you ever know you were my hero, and everything I'd like to be, I could fly higher than an eagle, you are the wind beneath my wings"--my son, my teacher, Danny. Even with the help of a pill, I choked, had to pause to get the words out. Tears were not only in my eyes but in the eyes of many of the women there who had followed Danny's progress over the years. Danny, unaffected by it all, stood and waved to the entire room. He truly was my hero, and I was not yet through learning from him.

We had every weekend filled for the next six weeks--the estate sale; followed by a garage sale; Doug's birthday; graduation; my National Convention and campaign in Denver, Colorado; and one weekend to pull it all together, as well as a family trip to Atlanta, Georgia.

Danny's little red truck came in handy as we had emptied grandma's house and moved it into every spare inch of mine. Putting mom in a nursing home had not been an easy decision, but she needed 24-hour care. The second broken hip was not one she was willing to work hard to overcome. She was 90 years old, she'd been independent, and she seemed to rather enjoy having people wait on her. We suspected that TA's were occurring as she had not only become incontinent but this grand lady, who, weeks before at age 90, would have told you to the penny the last five checks she wrote, or exactly what she'd eaten the Sunday before; lost track, couldn't remember, and grew increasingly dependent. Was she entitled? I think so. Did I like it? No. I had grown to love her over the years and had heard her say so often, "I hope I never lose my faculties, and I hope I can live alone until I die". After all these years of doing just that, of giving to people and to her family, to have her mind taken away seemed so unfair. I'd had eight years now to deal with the intricacies of the human mind as I watched Danny struggle to regain control; and I was now watching grandma give up. We were losing the part that had made her unique and unlike anyone else--the essence of what is each one of us--the words, thoughts, and ideas that can never die. I silently mourned her loss for her. Blessing or not, she was not very aware by now of those losses, nor had made the decision on her own to move ahead of me in her own secret mourning process to the acceptance stage.

One thing that never changed was her love for Danny, and her daily prayers for his recovery. Early in Danny's recovery, after he could chew, he had let grandma know that he really enjoyed M&M's, and they helped keep him going. From that day on, every week until her first fall during his senior year, grandma brought Danny a bag of M&M's. It wasn't just her weekly ritual that kept us smiling, but it was grandma's always frugal nature that had kept her in funds. She would do without something she really wanted because she was afraid she'd outlive her money. There was no convincing her otherwise and history has proven her to be correct. But no expense was to be spared when it came to the M&M's. Every Sunday, Danny got a one pound bag. Now he returns the favor.

It was graduation weekend. Tables were set up around the pool. I'd ordered hundreds of dollars in food to be picked up right after church that Sunday. All the other snacks, drinks, and party paraphernalia was in bags and boxes in the laundry room, ready to be put out and devoured.

It wasn't until I had picked Danny up from rehearsal and saw him walking toward me carrying his cap and gown, that the reality of what was occurring really hit me. If you stay busy enough to stay ahead of those thoughts that bring pain (although it may not be a very emotionally healthy thing to do) I'd been doing it for so long now that it wasn't often I let myself feel the pain. All smiles, Danny came towards me. He was graduating with his class. How proud he was. The tears began again, but I blinked them back while trying to keep the conversation light, determined not to spoil this celebration for Danny.

As I wrote a check that night for church the next morning, it really hit home what I'd known before; June 10, 1990, eight years to the day, that one split second which had changed how we would think, act, or say up to this very moment. Eight years to the day; we had done it--Danny was to graduate! He was now six feet tall and had become a thoughtful, loving, caring young man. Although he was still working to overcome the physical deficits, when his score was tallied as a human being, I couldn't find any there and I'm not sure the physician who had initially recommended life in a nursing home could have found any either. As a door closes, other doors open. We lose one of our senses; others grow stronger to help us compensate. We lose a talent and are often given even more important ones. And sometimes they're even given to a young man who's willing to share them patiently with a weepy mother. Right up to the graduation ceremony I found myself crying off and on for no real reason, although I suspect that somewhere my unconscious knew.

Seated directly in front of the staging area and next to the aisle, we watched as the graduates marched by to take their positions at the front of the school gym. Danny smiled as he came by, and I cried again. The tan linen dress I'd chosen for the ceremony was not a good choice; tears that fall on linen show up. It was only the beginning. Speakers addressed the graduates and families. I thought of how far the little boy, with tubes going in and tubes coming out, being kept alive by a respirator, looking so small in the big hospital bed, had come. Tears intermittently rolled down my cheeks. They were now going to sing the class song, "You are the Wind Beneath My Wings". I almost lost it. How ironic, I'd used that for Danny with no idea it would be the class song. But how very appropriate for this day, even though it now opened an emotional floodgate that I was having an awful time trying to control. Doug held my hand. I'm sure, even though he didn't show it on the outside, his heart was being racked by the same emotional tidal wave.

Students were called forward alphabetically to receive their diplomas. As one reached the stairs descending the platform, the next student was stepping on for their moment in the spotlight. The rehearsals had obviously been successful because it was amazingly smooth through the G's and into the H's.

"Daniel James Hoppe".

Danny stepped up to the platform, the applause started. The applause continued. He received his diploma. The applause continued. You could hear the whistles and sounds only teenagers make. Danny descended the platform.

The applause continued, not to stop until he was seated next to the previous graduate. Doug and I looked at each other, both of us feeling the warmth of those students and families throughout our small community who had watched Danny overcome obstacle after obstacle and still remained the smiling, caring young man he is today. So many of them had encouraged Danny in their special ways and followed his achievements that were food for articles in our small local newspaper, and they never once failed to respond. The people and businesses in this community of ours not only spoke verbally, but they spoke the greatest language of all--the language of love.

Graduation ceremonies over, the whole Hoppe clan filed out of the auditorium. After handshakes and doing our share of congratulating, which we felt to be insignificant after what our hearts had just received, we headed home for a graduation party that would go on until the wee hours of the morning. We had passed another milestone in Danny's recovery, and it was time for all of us to take a few weeks to just enjoy that and gear up for the college experience.

To everything there is a season,
and a time to every purpose under
the heaven:

A time to be born, and a time to
die; a time to plant, and a time to
pluck up that which was planted;

A time to kill, and a time to heal;
a time to break down, and a time to
build up;

A time to weep, and a time to
laugh; a time to mourn, and a time to
dance;

A time to cast away stones, and a
time to gather stones together; a time
to embrace, and a time to refrain
from embracing;

A time to get, and a time to lose; a
time to keep, and a time to cast away;

A time to rend, and a time to sew;
a time to keep silence, and a time to
speak.

A time to love, and a time to hate;
a time of war, and a time of peace.

Ecclesiastes 3:1–8

1990 CANDIDATE NATIONAL VICE-PRESIDENT 126

This year is a celebration of 50th year.

Fifty years brings to mind the word TRADITION. Tradition expresses what is. We are informed by our traditions and we are reformed by their impact upon us and by our faithful response to them. As tradition is the handing on of something to one's successor we must continue to strive to keep alive those qualities which were and are uniquely

We cannot disown what we have been. We need to not only own but recall the traditions, the ideals upon which was founded. As we look to define who we are maybe out of love and respect for our predecessors we should let traditions walk with us as we move forward.

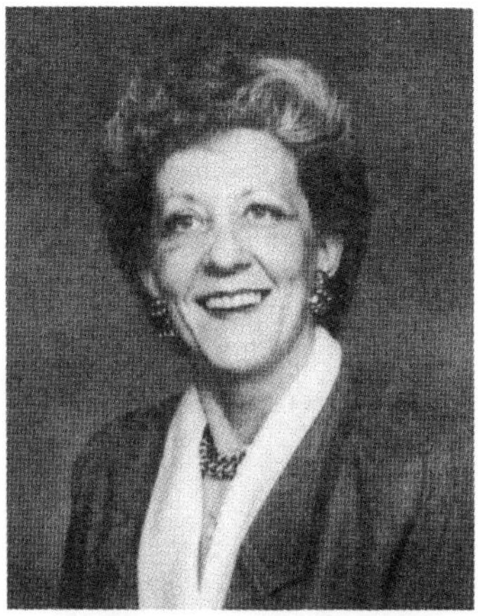

Those who would move us into the future must keep looking backward and then respond and reshape those traditions only so they work with today's members, not try and do away with them. For if we do, we sever our connection with the past and dilute traditions for those new members of tomorrow.

VOTE for HOPPE

VOTE for CHANGE

A CHANGE THAT MAKES SENSE

Life means to have something definite to do, a mission to fulfill. And in the measure in which we avoid setting our life to something we make it empty. Human life, by its very nature, has to be dedicated to something.

--José Ortega Y Gasset

CHAPTER 12

Graduation was on Sunday; the house returned to normal, laundry done, food purchased to refill an empty refrigerator, my campaign materials boxed for flight, my bags packed and that Thursday I boarded a flight for Denver, Colorado-- and another benchmark in my life.

Denver, the site of the 1990 Insurance Women's Convention. I was running for National Vice-President, vying for a spot on the Executive Board and daring to skip the Secretary position the "Way It Was ALWAYS Done"! I had prepared a brochure which reflected my beliefs, credentials and recommendations obtained from a myriad of industry and professional people, which I had mailed to insurance women all over the country. In two extra suitcases, I carried 800 brochures and chocolate coins wrapped in gold foil. ($90.00 in excess baggage fees.) I was prepared to WIN!

I've never been a relaxed flyer, but I'm not a white-knuckle flyer either. The skies were clear and the smooth flight let me lay back in the seat and do a review of the past weeks, months, and years, which kept my mind off the fact that I was 35,000 feet above the ground.

There was certainly no way to declare the past eight years had been a wonderful experience, because they hadn't. In my mind, the day Danny was hit was the yardstick by which I measured everything else. That was to me the one single, worst experience of my life. If whatever came into my life in the future didn't measure up to that pain, it just couldn't be that bad, and if it weren't that bad, then we'd get through it. I knew and had known that as long as I never had to stand next to a hospital bed or watch one of our six children, or one of my beloved grandchildren, fight for life, nothing could be that bad--absolutely nothing. So many things had been brought into perspective for me over the years when it came to what really mattered in my life. Although I believed I held a healthy perspective, I was still trying to fill every day with as much as I could put into 20 hours. Sleep--someday I'd sleep a long time--had to use every moment, even though so much of the pain had been solved by Danny's accomplishments. I still mourned for him, those things which had meant so much to him, that he probably would never have an opportunity to even try his beloved baseball. But over the past eight years, I had so firmly entrenched myself in the fast-paced, always busy, lifestyle that even when I tried to slow down, the rest was only a temporary one because I just kept saying "yes" until I filled it back up again. I could do it all.

Hadn't I shown everyone over and over again how well I could handle everything? The certificates on my office wall, the plaques, the letters of thank you, the education courses completed which resulted in letters after my name. Designations that represented study, not more income, were regarded by many as achievement, and, oh, was I an achiever.

When Doug had his heart problem, more than once I said to him, "You don't need to die for the company. You gave them 30 years at 100%--now back off. Don't let them hold that carrot in front of the horse, let the new guys have the trips, the watches, the damn coffee cups. If we want something, we can buy it."

Sounded so reasonable as it came out of my mouth, and so ridiculous when it entered my ears. Helen Reddy recorded a song several years ago, "I Am Woman, I Am Invincible". I was, and certainly nothing was ever going to happen to me. At least not for the next fifteen or twenty years. There was too much to do. And I also had the best argument in the world. When you could do something, and God gave you an ability or talent, weren't you supposed to use it? Wasn't it given to you, not for you, but to do for others or for His glory? Weren't we not risking losing by not using? I really believed that in my heart. But the unhealthy part was I was also using it to run away yet again from really confronting the initial pain of Danny's accident and Doug's pain that I hadn't been able to comfort. Pain that was now set aside became blown out of proportion by the effort I put into keeping it in its cubicle. I couldn't see then the destructiveness of not bringing it out and placing it in its proper perspective. I'd read self-help books, business books, people books, and had several hundred dollars worth of cassettes that promised to help you sell, negotiate, get motivated, change your attitude, learn forgiveness, make a difference, and find yourself. I had the answers. At least the ones I wanted. Doug had often said that our children came to us seeking advice and frequently accepted it only when it was what they wanted to hear. Well, I couldn't be put in the same category as the children, I never asked his advice.

I called home that first night in Denver, and Danny answered the phone. "Remember, Mom, you gotta want it, and you gotta want it bad. Give 'em hell, Mom, you can do it. Dad and I are rooting for you " were his parting remarks as he passed the phone to his father.

Doug came through also waving my banner, even though I knew he could care less about this agenda I had created. He, once again, supported me by faith, and I jumped into the battle with both feet. I could sleep when I got home as I made the caucuses and answered questions (off the cuff, which was a new and very enlightening experience). I was bucking the system, and some women let me know that in no uncertain terms.

I'd fall in bed only to arise three hours later, feeling pretty heated up. Judith Brilles has written about women sometimes being other women's worst enemies when they cross over and invade a comfort zone. For many it isn't saucers and milk time, it's time for the claws to start sprouting. I was making waves and enjoying every minute of it. I lost the race by a much narrower margin than I had anticipated, but losing didn't feel bad. As a matter of fact, it felt pretty good, because I could relax, shake hands, and go home much wiser from a political standpoint and much richer from having an opportunity to get to know so many more women who worked within the industry I loved and believed in. For all those who beat me up, there were many more who upheld me through the new friendships and that special caring only a woman can bring into a relationship. Sorry I lost? Oh, no. The only real losers in life are those who fail to try, who fail to follow through on a commitment.

Packing to come home was much easier, and unneeded luggage was packed in the larger ones. Being tired helps flights go faster especially when you're asleep.

> If I had a formula for bypassing trouble, I would not
> pass it around.
> Trouble creates the capacity to handle it.
>
> I don't embrace trouble;
> that's as bad as treating it as an enemy.
>
> But I do say meet it as a friend, for you'll see a lot of
> it and had better be on speaking terms with it.
>
> --Oliver Wendell Holmes

> Personally I'm always ready to learn, although I do not always like being taught.
>
> --Winston Churchill

CHAPTER 13

Once home, since I was not going to be a national officer, I could continue on the church boards, hold three chairmanships for the Insurance Women's Association, do their bulletin, attend head injury meetings, get Danny enrolled in college courses, tie up all the loose ends on my mother-in-law's house, arrange for a mortgage to build a church parsonage, do all the setup for a white elephant sale at the church, and start taking a parliamentary procedures class to become a registered parliamentarian. Piece of cake! I was also planning three trips out-of-town for September and October, which were fast-arriving.

I had promised my family that once the convention in Denver was over, I would really try to quit smoking. So off to my friendly G.P. I went and said, "I promised I'd do this; I need drugs." Having read once again about the successes that had been had with a blood pressure medication on affecting the pleasure center of the brain and reducing the craving for nicotine, I wanted that and

Valium to keep me from becoming this banshee that I knew I could be from past attempts. I also wanted a Stress Test and a breathing evaluation for a baseline. I knew that seeing concrete improvement would help keep me off if I eliminated those awful things that made my closet smell bad, cost me big bucks, and Danny hated. I vowed not to smoke in my office. I hadn't picked up my phone without a cigarette in my hand in 20 years, but I would do it. There was also no more smoking in the house. If I really wanted one, I had to do it outside. That became a little reminiscent of when I was a teenager. Although our folks knew we were smoking, it was absolutely not allowed in their presence, and we would go outside--rain or snow--and smoke (those cigarettes we had hoarded) under the old apple tree because even at twenty-five cents a pack, they didn't come easy.

My stress test was wonderful. I returned to a resting heart rate and blood pressure right on cue, just like a healthy person. The breathing test showed my air exchange was good, and there was very little tissue damage--they were surprised at that one. Yes, quitting now was the thing to do. Don't you always quit while you're ahead? Made sense to me. But there was no cold turkey, I couldn't do that. I did try but then decided I would limit them and stick to all the other rules and tried to put myself in non-smoking situations as much as possible. I discovered I just liked lighting them and having one in my hand. I bought the fake ones to hold. I was now down to three a day. Of course, I switched to the 120's, but it was only three a day; and only when I really, and I mean <u>really</u>, wanted one. My friend Carole, who had seen me through so many things the past ten years, sent me little notes of encouragement and congratulations for the effort. She had given me an owl once which held a little sign that said, "Please don't smoke", and I had that facing me at my desk. Danny liked not having it in the house and made his comments. We were going to overcome this thing.

I even managed to attend an Insurance Women's Fun Weekend in Ohio where there are "blue rooms" and only smoked one pack. I was doing great, for me! I also found that when you didn't stop for a cup of coffee and a cigarette, you could get more done. I was really on a roll now. Not only did I have my old standby, "the adrenalin rush", but nervous energy to keep me moving on life's roller coaster at breakneck speed. Doug started in again with his pleas to slow down.

"I can't right now; I've made all these commitments I can't back out of, no new ones," I promised.

September 19, 1990. The day began at 8:00 a.m. There were piles of folders on my desk, calls to be made regarding my upcoming trip to Indiana where my friend, Jan Kearbey, an insurance woman from Kansas, was flying into Detroit Metro. She and I would drive together to the state convention, and it all had to be coordinated. We finalized our plans, and I was looking forward to some time with this lady who made me laugh, who talked about endorphins and a healthy attitude and whose husband was terminally ill. She managed to practice what she'd preached to the other four who roomed together our year as Regional Vice Presidents. I knew I needed something to pep me up. Even Super-woman was feeling tired. I told Doug I wished I could get "just a little sick", not serious, so I could go to the hospital for a few days and rest. I was afraid I was burning out but couldn't or wouldn't just walk away from it, or admit to anyone else that the work-horse needed a break from the plow.

Trustee meeting that evening at church. The meeting was moving right along, the Pastor standing to my right. I don't remember the exact words, only the feeling I needed to respond to a statement. As I turned my head and looked up at him, my neck snapped, and an immediate pain hit my right temple. Boy, was it a pain, but it would pass. I didn't have time to be sick, not really. Trying to shake off the headache, I wrote notes and alternately rubbed my temple. The meeting over, I didn't stay for the usual visiting but took my cup of coffee and drove home. Boy, my head hurt. I had to get some aspirin and lay down. I was just going to bed.

As I shut the garage door and dropped my briefcase in its usual corner, Doug asked how the meeting went. "I don't want to talk about it now. I've got an awful headache. I'm going to bed." Nightgown on, two aspirins downed, I fell into bed. Doug made a trip up to check on me, put a cool cloth on my head and returned back downstairs to watch the rest of the TV show alone.

When he came up to go to bed himself, Doug tells me I got up. Dizzy, nauseous, and feeling even worse, I suggested to him that he should just cut my head off because the pain was so bad and proceeded to the bathroom where I vomited blood and fell unconscious to the bathroom floor.

I'm awake! The room was dimly lit; I was in a hospital bed. Well, wasn't this Wonderful; I'd finally snapped!. They had me on a psychiatric floor of a hospital. I'd gone to Indiana and had a nervous breakdown. Wonderful! Where was Jan, where were the other women? Obviously, Doug had to stay in Michigan and take care of Danny, so he couldn't be here at the hospital in Indiana. But why was I all alone and on the "nut" floor? I must have really done something!

It didn't occur to me then, or for days, that it was a physical illness. I couldn't be sick. I didn't have time. I'd seen Doug through lung problems, back surgery, open heart surgery; Danny the past eight years; grandma through eye surgery, stomach surgery, two broken hips; and all the other kids' mishaps. I didn't get sick physically. The two surgeries I'd had in my life were optional on my part. It couldn't be physical. I'd lost my mind; I knew it. They had me on this floor with other crazy people. I faded back into the velvet comfort of darkness.

I was awake again; the room was dim. Noises, people noises, groaning. Oh, the crazies, they were trying to kill me. I'm on the psycho floor, and they're trying to kill me. I'm all alone. Where is Jan? Where are my friends? I have friends in Indiana. Everyone is so nice in Indiana. Recalling the childhood trips there to visit relatives, I knew some of the best food in the world was in Indiana, but I didn't want to die there. They were trying to kill me, and I couldn't get out of this bed. They had me tied in. I was even more helpless and so scared. Oh, God, I'm scared! I have no control over this situation. I'm usually in charge, and now they're telling me what to do, and they've tied me in bed. I'm so scared! Floating in and out, I have no memory of sunshine for days. I only remember nights. I also have no memory of the respirator that sustained my life as it had done once before for Danny. I don't remember the feeding tubes or the monitors. The one that was inserted directly into my heart that I pulled out when they untied my hands, is only a scar by my collarbone--I don't remember it or wanting to remove it. But those days of intensive care and while on the regular floor are just an accumulation of brief periods of cognition. Once again, as my body produced adrenalin because of fear or anger, I rose high enough in consciousness to form a memory. Only when my body was reacting to the fight or flight response was I able to hold that memory.

My darling husband, who had supported me even when he thought I was wrong, was at my bedside almost round the clock. He had, once again, been thrown back into that ocean of hopelessness and helplessness that you find yourself swimming in as one you love lies near death. He had called 911 and waited that hour--which in reality was 15 minutes--until the paramedics arrived. He, once again, sat in the front seat of an ambulance, racing against time to the hospital Emergency. He sat, alone this time, and waited for news. Knowing in his heart that stress had brought this on, he blamed himself for not putting a stop to it sooner. Stress caused this, and, if I survived, he would never again allow me to live life in that fast lane of achievements, accomplishments, and ego. The world, Insurance Women, Head Injury, our church didn't need me out there trying to make a difference; but he needed me, and they would do without me in the future. And this time, I would not change his mind.

I hadn't lost my mind, only a small portion of it. CVA, Cerebrovascular Accident, a weakened blood vessel in the right frontal lobe had given out. Blood entered the brain and filled the right ventricle. The doctors would later say it stopped bleeding on its own, probably before the ambulance got there; but not knowing what caused it, or if it would happen again, they wanted more answers. Also, given my state of mind--what was left of it--I needed to be watched. Carefully.

In insurance, we call fires friendly and unfriendly. Friendly fires are those that stay within the confines which they were intended. On a cold winter evening, the flames dancing over logs in the fireplace feel warm and friendly. A hostile fire, on the other hand, is that spark that bounces out onto the carpet and flames head directly for your chair.

Blood does the same thing in the brain. When it remains in the arteries and veins, it brings life-giving oxygen to brain cells. When it escapes the confines for which it was intended, it wreaks havoc on the brain cells and the human thought processes. Injury to one area of the brain can cause swelling which can damage even remote areas of this lump of grey matter which makes us, each one of us, unique to the world and in the eyes of God. Mine (brain cells) were raging. They couldn't keep me tied in bed, someone was trying to kill me. I wanted away from all this, I wanted to go home. Please, oh, please, let me go home! On a

July day eight years earlier, hadn't I been told to take him home? Let him hear, see, smell familiar things that would be comforting and promote wellness. Hadn't Marilyn said that about Danny? Why weren't they taking me home to get well? Didn't anyone care? Was I that bad? And where was Marilyn? Where were my advocates? Hadn't I always been one for Danny, for Doug, for my uncle, my grandfather? Where the hell were mine? I was getting angry now; the fight response caused my old buddy adrenaline to course through my body. Pieces of memory began to become pieces of a puzzle. If they ask me one more time what kind of medicine they're giving me . . . "Decadron, you dummies, you're giving me Decadron. You put it in that little cup. Don't you know?" My God, what kind of people do they have taking care of me if I have to tell them what kind of medicine they're giving me? And, if they don't quit making me squeeze their fingers. That is just the dumbest thing. Why would a person who had lost her mind have to squeeze fingers? I'll squeeze your finger, and, if you ever untie me, I'm out of here. Boy, I thought the DWZ (Denver Women's Zone) of Denver was bad. This place is the pits. They're talking loud to me. I'm not deaf. Am I deaf? No. Then why are they in my face and talking so loud to me? Then they changed their tactics to moving their lips in an exaggerated fashion. "I'm not deaf, and I don't read lips either! Get away from me! I'm real mad now, and Doug is here." Well, isn't that great.

Finally Doug is at my bedside! Now, he's telling me I'm not in Indiana; I'm in Ann Arbor. I'm where? I don't remember leaving Indiana. The other faces are the same. How come I'm now in Michigan?

"Where are you, Sue?"

"I'm in Indiana."

"No, you're in Ann Arbor."

"No, I'm in Indiana."

How many hours or days I did this I don't know, but I knew I was in Indiana. Jan and I had been at the State Convention, and I went to "Flip City". I was in Indiana where the food was really good, and the cool things--ice cream, jello, milkshakes--felt good on my throat--which hurt. Had I been on a respirator? Why couldn't I remember that? Boy, the food tastes good, but then some of the best cooks in the world were in Indiana. I knew that.

"You're not in Indiana. You're in the hospital in Ann Arbor." Doug was angry; his voice had that same tone he used on the kids. Were his eyes red? Yes, they were that angry red we'd all accused him of. Of course, they didn't really get red, but the blaze of anger from them had always made that a good analogy.

"I'm not in Ann Arbor. The hospital is in the township anyway. I'm in Indiana." I'm really mad now. How dare he talk to me as if I were a child. Nice guy I married. Make me stay in this place and then come here and holler at me. Boy, was I lucky and am I mad now.

But the anger kept me awake and kept me thinking. I didn't fade out. Was he trying to tell me something without telling me something? Maybe our insurance wouldn't cover me if I were in Indiana, and he was doing something so it would be covered. Maybe I should say "Ann Arbor" so the bills would be paid. Doug loved me; I knew that. Never in 20 years had I ever had to question the love that he gave so unconditionally. I was an insurance person; he expected me to get the message. Oh, yeah! I got it!

"Where are you, Sue?"

"Ann Arbor."

"She's coming around" the nurse said.

They liked the answer. They were smiling. So was I-- inside. I knew I was in Indiana. I had fooled my captors. I was well enough; they were transferring me to Rehab. I was on my way, one step closer to going home.

In the safety of the rehab bed, I remembered the other hospital rooms in tiny confetti-like images. A huge man was holding me in his arms over a hospital bed. His voice so deep and assuring. He said, "Don't worry; I've got you. I won't let anything happen to you." For the first time I felt safe. I remembered that experience as being my moment of safety in that sea of fear raging around me. I felt secure for that period of time, while someone else in the same situation may have been terrified (of being lifted and suspended in the air).

I remembered another hospital room where I lay trembling from fear; they were trying to kill me. I knew I'd never get out of the hospital alive. A nurse named Kristin (I'll never forget her name; I even remember telling her I'd never forget her name because my best little friend in the world was an eight-year-old little girl from church named Kristin, and she and I were building a doll house, so I'd always remember her) knelt at my bedside and held my trembling body while they called for Doug to come back to the hospital. He came (I don't remember that), but Kristin kept me safe.

I remember another hospital room where they got me out of bed, raced me down the hallway and put me in a shower. It was early in the morning. I didn't shower in the morning; I didn't want to do this. And then I'm wet all over, and it's cold. I'm so cold; I'm shivering. Let me out of here; I didn't want a shower, and now I'm cold. Let me out of here. Water hitting me in the face, the nurse sprayed me in the face. Why would she do that? I was just cold. At the time it occurred, it startled and scared me. Better behave. Now that I felt safe, anger boiled near the surface. How dare she! Tell me on her shift I'd take a shower when she decided. I'll have Doug intercede and tell them no morning showers. How dare she!

Looking back, I don't remember what precipitated the face spraying. I don't remember being combative, but maybe I was. Maybe she thought it was one way to bring the situation under control. It sure did, but there had to have been a better way rather than instill fear and panic and now, anger.

I remember being tied in bed, tugging against the restraints. I remember climbing out of bed one time, somehow toppling all the IV poles. I remember the nurse who was very upset about that and my rising ire at being chided as though I were a child. Didn't these people know that I was an adult woman? I was a business woman. I wasn't a dummy; I wasn't deaf, I couldn't read lips, and I was certainly not used to being told what to do every waking moment.

Now I'm in Rehab where it's hard to walk. They shuffle me around in a wheelchair and expect me to remember how to get to all those other rooms when I'm not doing it myself, and they're treating me like I have brain damage. If I'm in Ann Arbor, where's Marilyn? Marilyn can help me. She talks their language. I'm saying all the things, but they are not listening to me. Nobody listens to me.

I'm in front of the mirror. There are marks that lay in a design from collarbone to collarbone that look like a necklace. Did they have IV's in my neck? Did they have me hooked up to monitors through my neck? Was I like Danny; did I have brain damage? Why couldn't I remember? The last clear memory was being at the church, pain in my head. I came home and went to bed. Then I was in Indiana. I remember the hospital in Indiana and then the other hospitals before I ended up back in Ann Arbor in rehab. What happened to me? Why don't I know what's going on? I'm always in control, always in charge. Aren't I the one who chairs the committees, runs the office, gets things done. Why won't they listen to me now?

I remembered tests; I remember them sending me down this tunnel; I remember going berserk when they tried one time to strap my head down--can't stand confining places--scared, out of control, panicked.

Solace in food. Food is good, and they bring me these milk shakes. Five a day. They feel so cool on my throat. Physical therapy now becomes the focus of my anger.

I had tried in vain to intimidate the head of the rehab program, whose innovative ideas and his caring for those lost in the nether world of brain damage guided him to establish a much respected TBI rehab unit. He came in for a visit. I threatened him with bodily harm if he didn't let me go home. He left the room, and I went to therapy.

Walking between parallel bars--now, isn't this stupid? I can walk. My God, I'm not a baby! See, I can walk. I bump into the sides. "This wouldn't happen if you'd give me my high heels back." Expect me to walk in these tennis shoes. "If you would just give me the 3-inch heels I've worn for 30 years, there wouldn't be a problem. Give them to me, I'll show you!"

"Find your way out of P.T., Sue. How do you get back to your room?"

"How should I know? You guys brought me here. I didn't check the door out when I came through it. It's your problem."

So this is what it's like when your brain snaps. Now, they're throwing a term around, "CVA". What the hell is a CVA? Someone else said stroke. I had a stroke? No, I've never been sick. I always take care of people. Aneurysm, now there's a word. Did I have one? No, people die from those; they don't live. I've known two people who died, and I'm alive. Aren't I alive? Yes, I'm alive. I'm in a hospital rehab unit. I have two doctors, "The Wonderful Dr. Wardner" and that other one, what's his name, oh, yes, Dr. "I want to be God" Thomas. He's the one who wants to shoot me down that drainage tile (MRI) again. No way. No more of those.

I want to see my grandbabies. Where are they? I remember C.J. was here. No, not here, other hospital. His mom snuck him into my room, he climbed into bed with me, and I cuddled him. He kept saying, "I love you, Nana" and fed me chocolate candy. He wanted me to get better. I'm getting better. Where are the rest of them? I want to go home! I <u>have</u> to go home!

> The art of medicine consists of amusing the patient
> while nature cures the disease.
>
> --Voltaire

CHAPTER 14

Standing in the archway of my kitchen, Doug and Danny are eating lunch as I calmly tell them there's something going on that I don't understand. Maybe I've really stretched myself so thin with all the 20-hour days, the committees, the church work, the Insurance Women, I've snapped. I know I've been checking myself in and out of hospitals, and they can't find any physical problems. Maybe it's time to go out to St. Joe Emergency and have them take a look. I'm getting worried about myself, and I am so tired all the time lately. I'd call later, kissed them goodbye. Briefcase in hand, I left the house, started up the van, pushed in a Wayne Dryer tape, and drove to St. Joe. They admitted me, put me in a private room. I'd be better now.

It was morning, and I was tipping my way down the parallel bars, and they wouldn't give me my heels back. Well, time to check out of here. When Doug got here, he could get my stuff together--the flowers, the cards, the stuffed animals (lots of sheep), and my clothes and carry them out to the van. I'm going home. Doug is standing in the doorway. No, I'm not going home. I'm sick, I need to stay right where I am.

"Like hell, I'll stay here. Give me my van keys. I know you took them out of my purse. It's my van; it's titled in my name. I own it. Give me the keys."

Doug said he didn't have the keys; the van was home.

"No, it isn't. I drove it to the hospital. I know exactly where it is in the lot. Won't give me the keys? Okay, I'll call the police." (I explained to the police woman what I wanted, not knowing that it was only the hospital switchboard that was intercepting my call. The police would get me out of here.)

I continued to yell at Doug. "I checked myself into this hospital; I'll check myself out. In the meantime, you think about it while I trash this room." I began, but soon I was face down on the bed. They are holding me down. Doug is helping. Why is he helping?

"You have a choice--take these pills or get a shot. Which do you want?" the nurse asked.

"If I have only those choices, give me the pills," I said in defeat. I'd lost again, and Doug was on their side. He didn't want me at home. He was afraid of me is why he didn't want me home. I was a nut case! But I'd taken care of him! All those months with his back, the home traction, the weeks in the hospital, the recovery. The trip where he could have died at any moment, the heart surgery, the recovery. I'd taken care of him! Now, he was too scared to take care of me. How dare he? I was mad again.

"Well, I've taken the pills, but I want you to know you've broken it. When I'm well, and I will get well and get out of here, the first stop is an attorney's office. I'm all done." I laid back on the bed. (Doug left the room to cry in a nurse's arms.) I was really mad now, really mad and really sleepy.

Only a few days' blur this time. There's to be a team meeting. Dr. Wardner will discuss how we're going to handle my case. I understand team meetings--I'd been having them for Danny twice a year for eight years. Some good, some bad; but I know what to expect. Sure I do!

We sat around a table and Dr. Wardner directed questions to each of the therapists. I could hear the tone of his voice change as he talked one to one with people around the table. Isn't that interesting? He changes his tone of voice with each person. How come I can hear that? I never have been able to pick up on voice inflections before. Doug always seemed to, but, somehow, I always missed it. How come now? This was so new, felt so strange. I'd have to store it away, needed to sharpen up and pay attention, was imperative I pay attention.

"Sue, you have to be very careful when you walk; a piece of paper could cause you to slip. Be sure to keep the floor of your room clean. If there is water, call someone in to clean it up."

"I'm to be a housekeeper now. For what it costs for that rehab bed, I'm supposed to be in charge of keeping it clean? My own alarm clock, get myself up for therapy? What am I paying you guys for?" The full realization of just how bad I'd been and the deficits I still had weren't registering. I never got sick.

Next on the agenda was an MRI. They wanted a good one, a complete look at my brain. I'd have to agree to being confined in that drain tile, endure that test, and they'd think about me going home. To get out of here, to go home, I'd do anything. Wasn't I tough? Hadn't I survived many things much worse than that? Wasn't it worth it if I could go home? Yes, I'd let them have their test. I'd grit my teeth, toughen up. I had to go home. Yes, I'd do the test.

I went back to my room, happier than I'd been in days. I'd do their test, and I could go home, where I could lay in my own bed at night, be cradled safe in Doug's arm, where body, mind and soul could heal. I could have a house full of noisy grandchildren, I could be with Danny, have my own things; I could run my hands over my things; I needed to touch them, every one of them. I would behave, I would do their test, and I'd go home--my home, that had taken on new value, a new meaning, and represented safety wellness.

Pastor's in my room visiting with me. He'd been there many times over the past few weeks, but I didn't remember that then, nor do I now, but he had been there. Now he was helping me fill out the form authorizing the MRI. We went through the questions. Did I have claustrophobia? Did I have problems with small confining places? You bet, but I'd get through it. I signed the forms, and they were whisked away by the nurse. Going to shoot me down that drain tile again. I'd do it this time, I'd stay in there for as long as they needed me to if it meant I could go home--had to go home.

Pastor left; I laid down and memories, pieces of memories, drifted back. I'm in this tunnel; I'm strapped down; I can't see my hands; and this glass so close to my face, can't be in here, let me out of here. They are about to put me in that tunnel, they want to strap my head down, I go berserk, can't do this. Now, I had signed a paper saying I could. Could I? Not sure, had to talk to the doctor. I got out of bed and went outside my room to the nurses' station.

"I need to talk to the doctor."

"Sorry, doctor's gone home for the day. Why don't you lay down and rest?"

Rest, they want me to rest. I can't do that test, I'm getting upset. I have to do it, but I'm getting scared. Have to get help. I'll call Doug, he bowls tonight. Looked up the number, they were paging him. What's taking so long? Can't wait. I'll call Marilyn, her recorder answered. Who could I call now? Needed help, needed a sedative, had to get myself under control, couldn't get out of control again, couldn't give into panic, was too close to going home. I'd ask for a sedative.

"Nurse, can I have a sedative? I know I'm blowing this test out of proportion. Can I have something?"

"No, you just lay down and relax."

Why won't they help me? What have I done that no one will help me? I'm losing control again; I'm scared. I hate being scared, but I am. Now, I'm crying; tears are pooling on the top of my hands. A nurse, dark hair and snappy black eyes, is standing near me.

"Mrs. Hoppe, you're going to have to pull yourself together," she said coldly and left the room.

Boy, she's full of compassion! Pull myself together? I'll pull myself together, and I'm out of here. I'm going home. One way or another, I'm going home. Grabbing my jogging outfit I go into the bathroom where I try to make myself presentable to the outside world. Can't go walking around the country looking like a wild woman. The hospital wrist band, can't get it off. It's got red on it. Doug said that meant "Watch this patient". Tucked it up in the sleeve. Had to look normal. Now, money, I needed money so I could buy a pack of cigarettes. Couldn't smoke in hospitals anymore, it might kill you. That was funny. Cigarettes might kill me, so they wouldn't let me smoke. But they put my life in danger before by having me on that psycho floor where they were trying to kill me, and they sent me down that tube where I could die, and they worry about cigarettes. And while I was thinking about cigarettes, how come, if they didn't want you smoking, how come they had pictures of them all over the place, on the wall of my room? There may have been a line through it, but it was my main visual focus from the hospital bed for weeks now.

I had gone from two, sometimes three, packs a day down to one a day before I came to the hospital. I almost had it licked. But as I focused on that cigarette, persevering, unable to get my thoughts off one, how I wanted just one drag. Please give me a cigarette. Take me outside for a cigarette. I'd kill for a cigarette. Well, now, I'd buy a whole pack and smoke them all. I was out of here. It's dark, it's late. Better find some I.D., too, so they can identify the body if I don't make it home. Tucked the small black letter case in the waistband, didn't want to look suspicious, walked out of my room, turned left, ended up at the wall with the pictures. Oh, this was the way to therapy, didn't want to go there, wanted the front door. I walked by the nurses' station, hit the button to open the unit doors and headed straight for the chapel. Had to go there first. Needed help and strength to get me home, had to go home. They wouldn't help me here, had to go home. That morning, I couldn't find my way out of the therapy room, but tonight I know exactly where I'm going.

Adrenalin is pumping, and I know exactly what I'm doing. No apprehension, no confusion, it's all clicking. Chapel first, and then home. I enter the tiny chapel. The lighted stain glass pictures bring instant comfort. Jesus with the children. Weren't we supposed to have the unquestioning faith of a child? Yes, I had that faith. Oh, God, I can't fall prostrate on the floor before you, there isn't enough room, but I will be there in my heart and mind. I am humbled before you. I give you my life. If I'm to die, there's too much left for me to do, but I'll go. If you don't want me now, then, please, put your hand under my arm and help hold me up. I can't stay here where they won't help me, I have to go home.

As I rose from the chair, there was a confidence that hadn't been there for weeks. I pushed open the chapel door, and I didn't go the wrong way. I went down the hall, into the lobby, and right out the front door, knowing exactly which way the road was that would take me out of the township and into town, and then how I would walk to get from Ann Arbor to Saline. If I had to walk the whole distance, I would.

Hold your head up! Walk purposely. Don't look like you're trying to hide anything. You're out for a fitness walk, move along. Wow! Look at me, loose gravel. I'm walking on loose gravel, and I'm not falling. Tell me I'll fall on a piece of paper, make me think I'm sick, and you, you dummy, you were believing them. You almost bought into all that "little Sue can't do anything".

Police--when they figure out I'm not coming back, they'll call the police. Can't walk right out here in the road, get over behind those bushes. Look at me, I'm walking on grass, on uneven ground, and I'm not tipping over, not falling. Hold me up, God. "Our Father", I prayed over and over as I walked the miles to where I could see the lights of the business district. There was a pond just off the road; my legs were getting tired. I'd been in bed a long time, how long I don't know. I didn't even know what month it was. How long had I been in the hospital? I had to rest.

I sat down next to the water, remembering a pond on my grandpa's farm where I'd caught frogs in the summer and ice skated in the winter. Some of my memory was still intact. The 23rd Psalm, learned in Sunday School so many years ago, was also stored in those long-term memory banks. "The Lord is my Shepherd", the verse, the water, the cover of darkness, the feeling of being in control of my life again was comforting. God would hold me up 'til I got home, then I'd be safe, then I'd decide what was going to happen to me. No more panic. Sue was back in control, and I would stay in control. I was not going back to that hospital. I'd scream, cry, threaten, maybe even take drastic measures. I was not going back.

I had been surviving in the hospital, existing in a bubble of fear and uncertainty. This same fear had immobilized me as a child as I lay in my bed, terrified as my stepfather ranted and raved at my mother, threatening to kill us all. What we learn in childhood often becomes the garbage that we carry along with us for years and years. While I was afraid and uncertain, I could do nothing. With the rush of anger came the motivation to change my situation. I began to operate then outside the fear-led approach. The witch doctor or voodoo priest who control their believers by fear were right up there with those in the medical profession who had saved my life during those foggy days of half consciousness.

No longer paralyzed by fear, next to the calming water, I gave it up completely as I said, "I shall fear no evil." "Let go and let God", another phrase I'd heard often in church took on new meaning. I was letting go, and I was going home. Well, God, grab hold; we've got a ways to go. Up the bank, back onto the road. Sheriff's Department is up ahead on the left. By now, the hospital has called them. I'll walk in back of the office building so I won't stand out. I can cut through the restaurant parking lot and come out at the signal. If I'm a jogger, have to look like one. Push the button, jog in place, don't call attention to yourself. The wheels are turning; I can think again; I can plan; I can remember the events of the evening, all of them, no gray areas. My legs were very tired by the time I crossed that intersection. Eight more miles. Could I go eight more miles? No, I had to call someone to come and get me. Money--couldn't spend money on a call, saving that for cigarettes. Didn't need money, I knew my calling card number. I knew my number.

Numbers had been plaguing me for days. I'd ask Doug, "When will you be back?" He'd tell me, and then I couldn't remember. I finally started spelling out the time, f-o-u-r-t-h-i-r-t-y, or whatever he said. I could remember a number if I made it a word. All the years of therapy with Danny sure came in handy in developing compensatory strategies. But if I couldn't remember numbers, how come I knew that phone number? Well, it didn't matter. At least, I didn't have to spend any of my cigarette money. Had to pick the right spot for the call.

Red Lobster, I'd go to the Red Lobster. The phones were by a window where I could see out. Yes, that's where I'd go. Phone in hand, it occurred to me I hadn't really thought about whom to call. I'd been praying in my room as I got dressed, "God, please send David, please send David." Knowing that David was the son who was most likely to bend to my will, I wanted him to come, but he hadn't. While walking, I'd prayed for someone from the church to come by, knowing they would take me home first, ask questions later, but they hadn't come either. Well, they may have, but I was walking behind bushes and buildings. How were they supposed to see me? Can't pray and ask for something and then play hide and seek. Think . . . who? Skip, I'll call Skip (Callie's husband), my son-in-law built like a Paul Bunyan reincarnated. We had a good relationship, and I adored their little boys. I'd call Skip; I remembered his number.

"Skip, I'm at Red Lobster. I need you to come pick me up. My legs are getting so tired. I'm afraid I'll fall in front of a car. Will you come?"

He hesitated. I didn't know until later that he hesitated because he was thinking, sure she's at Red Lobster. She's been in Indiana, why not the Red Lobster!

I read the pause as his plan to bring a posse, and my brain started running through options. The flight response kicking in full force.

"Sure, I'll come and get you. Let me get my dad to stay with the boys, and I'll be there as soon as I can."

Hanging up the phone, I knew that I had to get out of the building where they could trap me. That wild animal feeling, like when Doug held me down at the hospital, came back. Hide. I'd hide and make sure he came alone. There were shrubs in front of a car where I could sit and see the front door of the restaurant. I'd wait there. If he came alone, I'd come out. If not, well, it would be "So long, folks". I was not going back to that hospital.

So hide I did, hoping the people who owned this big car would savor their dinner, have a drink, visit, anything but leave before I knew what my next step would be. A car was pulling up in front; Skip was getting out, going in. I'd check the car; he was alone. As he came out of the restaurant, I took his arm. I'm sure he was surprised I was there. I could have been at the hospital writing another script in my head, but I wasn't; and we needed to get out of here; and I really wanted a cigarette now that I was beginning to relax.

We were moving. My legs were grateful they weren't the powering force. The car seat felt good. I felt good. I tried to convince Skip that I wouldn't tell anyone he came and got me.

But he said, "Somehow, I'll be in trouble anyway, so might as well be in for the whole thing. You're coming to our house."

"Okay, but I need to stop at the store and get some cigarettes."

We stopped. Skip went in and got them, and in twenty minutes I was drinking real black coffee, smoking a cigarette, and had three little boys climbing all over me. Nana was having the best time she'd had in weeks. Their little soft, fat arms around my neck were better than any medicine the doctor could have given me. They were life, the promise of tomorrow. And like my grandfather, so dear to me, who has lived forever in my memories, they were the promise that my spirit would live on long after the body gave way to time. What a blessing they were, how thankful I was becoming for the small joys I had often taken for granted. I would never do that again. Never be too busy again.

Even feeling so good, back in control of my life again, I knew I had to go home and tell Doug I was home to stay. Whether he was scared of me or not, whether he liked it or not. As it turned out I didn't need to go home to confront Doug, he was coming through the front door, our Pastor right behind him.

"What do you think you're doing? You have to go back to the hospital." All six feet, 190 pounds of him, by body language said, "And I'm going to see to it."

"I'm not going back to the hospital, not back to where they won't help me. And you're not taking me anywhere." Anger raged. How dare he suggest that!

"Let me hug you, hold you," he asked.

"You stay away from me; don't touch me. I'm not going back to the hospital. You don't seem to understand, they wouldn't take care of me, and I'm not going back."

Our Pastor was busy trying to find an answer, a compromise to the battle that raged. David pulled into the driveway. Callie went out, and they argued outside as to what was best for Mom. Three little boys watched the adults, each struggling to win the battle, keep talking for their wants, not stopping to listen. Pastor finally called the doctor who had himself been dealing with the staff at the hospital who had let me walk away. My daughter-in-law, David's wife, worked for a local head injury rehabilitation program, and she had also taken the hospital staff to task for not monitoring me.

I had prayed for David to come to the hospital as I dressed that night, prayed as I walked down the halls. "Please send David." But as I came back into my usual operating mode, the impatience that had always plagued me couldn't wait for the prayer to be answered. David was in my room probably about the same time I walked out the front door. He had searched the hospital, called another church member who had helped us with grandma Hoppe to see if she knew where his Dad might be. She, in turn, had called the church where a meeting was going on, which soon turned into a search party. The answer to another prayer. But I was, by then, asking for them, but also hiding behind bushes and buildings. When I prayed and asked God for things, I wanted them right now! And he could hunt for me to give them to me. At least, that's the way it looks to me as I look back on that evening.

Doug arrived at the hospital about the same time as Pastor, and the troops were out scouring the roads between the hospital and Saline. Skip had called our daughter, Denise, just to let her know where I was in case someone called her. They did, and she told them where I was. Now, they were in my face telling me I was going back to the hospital. Over my dead body! And they weren't sure it might not be.

The doctor was going to let me stay home for the night. There was no point upsetting me further. I could stay home and call him in the morning. Pastor had calmed the raging storm. I could sleep in my own bed--for one night--sleep in my own bed.

I had been committed to winning that battle. I had stayed committed long after the mood in which I had made the commitment left me. I'd won! I was on the road back. I knew it. Once again, I'd gotten mad, gotten determined, and won. I was getting well. I was going home.

As I walked into my house, it really was my house. For the first time in our married life, for Doug had owned this house when we got married, it was my house. I was home, and I touched things--the table of inlaid wood made by Doug's great uncle by hand, that stood in our entry. I'd rescued that table, paid good money to keep it in the family for one of our sons. My table, my house, my bedroom. The king-size bed that we'd shared for 20 years, where Danny was conceived, lay in welcome. When I was finally ready for bed, I fell into the comforting softness as parts of my body, in contact with the mattress, remembered.

Doug's arms were around me. Not afraid of him now, I clung to him, safe in his arms, safe in his love. I was home. I had no memory of the nights he held me in the hospital, saying silent prayers for me to get well, for me to be Sue again--not the pitiful, scared, pleading woman he often encountered, or the one out of control who couldn't remember. "Please, God, give me Sue back."

Later, I was to tell him that you have to be careful what you pray for, and then be ready when you get it. For that night, Sue came back with all the determination and hard charging nature that had driven me for forty-seven years. Sue was back and laying in the warmth and safety of his arms in my bed, at peace for the first time in weeks, really at peace.

His hand was moving over my body. Felt good, I was enjoying it. We were making love; I hadn't even thought about that. Must have forgotten that, too. Why hadn't I thought about that? It had been a real part of our married life. How could I have forgotten. I quit thinking about it, caught in the moment. And when it was over, wept in Doug's arms, overcome. But the emotion of an act which I'd also taken for granted for so long, forgetting the beauty, the wonder, the joy of passion when it's right. I was safe. I was home.

When things go wrong, as they sometimes will,
When the road you're trudging seems all uphill,
When the funds are low and the debts are high,
And you want to smile, but you have to sigh,
When care is pressing you down a bit--
Rest if you must, but don't you quit.

Life is queer with its twists and turns,
As every one of us sometimes learns,
And many a fellow turns about
When he might have won had he stuck it out.
Don't give up though the pace seems slow--
You may succeed with another blow.

Often the goal is nearer than
It seems to a faint and faltering man;
Often the struggler has given up
When he might have captured the victor's cup;
And he learned too late when the night came down,
How close he was to the golden crown.

Success is failure turned inside out--
The silver tint of the clouds of doubt,
And you never can tell how close you are,
It may be near when it seems afar;
So stick to the fight when you're hardest hit--
It's when things seem worst that you mustn't quit.

--A Winner

> Honor a physician with the honor due unto him for the uses which ye may have of him: for the Lord hath created him.
>
> --Ecclesiasticus

CHAPTER 15

Morning came too soon. The doctor was on the phone. He'd call back in two hours and talk to me about when I'd be back to see him. Doug suggested I crawl from the warmth and safety of my bed and get up to face the day ahead. I could do that. This time it would be on my terms. I got up.

By the time I talked to the doctor on the phone, I had put on my navy blue "power" suit, nylons, my 3-inch navy heels, my jewelry and my makeup. I was ready for business, and I told him that. I'd also be there at 1:00 to talk to him.

My wonderful Dr. Wardner heard my words and humored me. Life was going to be good again. I felt in control again. It would be okay. I was going back to the hospital on my terms, looking like me, walking like me, and thinking like I hadn't been about to think for weeks. The anger had cut through the fog created by the aneurysm. I was, by no means, fully recovered but I was back in charge and the panic was gone.

We parked the car in the hospital parking lot and walked hand in hand back into the Rehab unit. I wasn't off balance, and there was purpose back in the stride of the woman who pushed open the double doors. The difference in me became apparent in the looks on the nurses' faces. My regular day nurse greeted me, arms outstretched, soon to enfold me and welcome home the lady who went to dinner at Red Lobster. I had created a number of conversations the past 16 hours and would probably be the topic for many more. Word travels fast in a hospital.

Marilyn, who had spent unremembered hours at my bedside, came to my rescue once again as we negotiated my return to rehab. Now that some reason had replaced fear and my memory was beginning to hold its own, she suggested that I be allowed to visit the lab where the MRI was to be done and talk to the technician before the test so I could feel more comfortable. They would not strap my head, and,now that I was more in control, they would not strap my hands. I would have a hand buzzer, and,if I just couldn't stand it, they would get me out of there. They also promised that they would give me drugs--lots of drugs, guaranteed to keep me relaxed. Okay, I'd do the test, stay at the hospital, resume therapy. This time my trip home had been a real one. This time I truly made the decision to be admitted, but I had only gone about three steps up the wellness stairway. There were many more ahead.

Back in the hospital I now got up in the morning, put on a suit and my high heels, and went to therapy. My physical therapist, after putting me through the parallel bars, the steps, the side steps (called braiding), decided that just plain walking would be good for me. So I was assigned a friendly, cheerful fellow named Marvin to walk me around the medical complex, trying to get me lost, making me retrace my route, working as much with my mental, as my physical health. His cheerful spirit and friendly smile never failed to set my mood for the day. We walked; I got lost; I struggled; but every day, it got better.

One morning we were going down one of the endless, windowless, maze-like halls of the complex when I saw a sign. The name was the same as my head injury support group newsletter that I had written for so many years. Instantly ready to do battle, I said, "I'm going in here."

"No, we need to go back" he said.

"No, not until I find out what they do." I'm not sure if I were so much curious as I was testing the water again, as to who was in control.

Well, I asked and was told that they were the patient relations department of the hospital, and they were there to listen to complaints. Boy, did I have complaints. I wanted to see someone in my room at 1:00 that afternoon. I asked for it, and I got it. Poor lady had to sit through quite a few complaints before I got to the praises for the quality of the rehab department, even though the little nurse who had so callously passed off my fear the night I left the hospital could have jeopardized the whole program if anything had happened to me. I certainly wasn't a famous person but I knew a lot of people and the lawsuit that could have resulted could have created even more problems. How good it felt to talk and feel like people were really listening again. But even better, I could remember what I said and what they said. Well, maybe not right after, but I was beginning to be aware that things were moving from short-term memory to long-term memory by themselves. Ten minutes after the fact, I had a problem. Four or five hours, or if you could wait 'til the next day, I'd remember. Sure made for some long pauses in a conversation.

The other thing that began was the growing determination that, given the fact I had survived this insult to my brain, I was going to approach life not only with a new perspective, but also a sense of humor. Hadn't Jan been telling me for months about laughter creating endorphins that not only made you feel better but kept you healthy. I'd read the book, heard the tapes on Norm Cousins. Wasn't there a university in California that was investing a lot of money to do a study on this? Hospitals were even beginning to recognize that laughter might be the best medicine. I was going to take getting well seriously but everything else a whole lot lighter. I figured if something were not going to matter 10 years , well, five years even a year from now, I was not going to waste 15 seconds on it. I began to have fun with people for real, the first time in years. The people were fun; the work was not.

In Occupational Therapy, they made me plan a meal, go to the grocery store and buy the necessary foods, and then we played "Let's find the car in the parking lot". Because it was red, it was pretty easy--my brown van would cause me concern often later on. I even had to invite Doug to the hospital for lunch. It wasn't bad enough to have to cook, I had to let him know I could do it. They wouldn't let me keep it a secret. I'd never enjoyed cooking before except on holidays when all the family was around. The rest of the time, if it weren't canned or frozen, it didn't touch anything in my kitchen. I had often hoped they would have a fund raiser for a group who were really trying to develop the breakfast, lunch and dinner pills that could be taken and cooking and dishes could be eliminated completely. I planned; I cooked; I kept organized in a strange kitchen. Gave my therapist a quick in-service on the proper way to set the table, and Doug ate it and survived. No more cooking, whew!

My speech therapist, who came very highly recommended to me by one of the past patients, a young man at that time in therapy with Danny, had run the gamut with me. I knew just enough of the terminology to be a real pain.

One day, as I sat down to begin another session, she said, "Sue, this is what we're going to do; this is what we're looking for; this is what we hope to gain. So, can we just get to work with no questions?"

A little knowledge may not hurt you, but it sure does play havoc sometimes with people who are trying to help. But we laughed a lot, too. I would point to my right temple and refer to the big bang of 1990 and refused to let the failures make me depressed or feel sorry for myself. With the ability to retain more and more from day to day, I began to tie into even more of the long-term memories of Danny that I hadn't thought about for years. Marilyn said I had done that earlier, so I kept directing my treatment by saying, "Marilyn says". The wonderful Dr.

Wardner had become increasingly angry with her until they had a conversation where it was made clear to him that I was, in fact, retrieving old knowledge and applying it to what I thought my situation was and tagging onto it "Marilyn says". Sure am glad she was and is my friend, even though I did get her in a little trouble.

Now that I was really mobile on my own, I also went outside at intervals and smoked. I'd tell them at the nurses' station and take my friendly little watcher (who now sat outside my room 24 hours a day) with me. Some were delightful with their own stories to tell; others just were. But I had my business clothes back, and people acted like they cared about what I thought or felt or wanted, so who cared? It was now getting to that time in fall when the sun still shown brightly on the now colored leaves on the trees but did not provide much warmth, at least to most people. My aides would sit with me with their jackets on and shiver at times; I no longer was cold. My hands and feet, for most of my life were cold from September to May and, at any given time, the other four months. Now I was warm all the time. Not only had my attitude been adjusted but so had my body thermostat. When it got even cooler, they watched me out a window. Why would I want to run away now? I was somewhat in control. I moved around almost as I pleased, and I had cigarettes to smoke and plenty of new people everyday outside to talk to.

"Maybe I can help some family while I'm here", I remember thinking one morning. Doug and I had counseled with any number of new families the past eight years as regards living with head injury. I'd visited new families in this hospital. So I was here, might as well do what I can. I didn't go prowling around the hospital looking for them, but there was a father there with his head-injured son; a father and daughter waiting for mom who had had her own CVA--they were calling her's a stroke--to come around. We talked several times. Drawing from my own fear-led emotions of those first two weeks, I encouraged them to keep reassuring, to be near her as much as possible, maybe even arrange with the nurse to allow them to be just verbally more demanding as regards their mother's care so that maybe she would sense on some level that there was someone there watching over her from outside the medical profession. I had written my own script. We didn't know she wasn't doing the same thing. Maybe she had gone to Indiana also--hope she enjoyed the food there as much as I did.

Speaking of food, I had enjoyed the food so much my skirts were tighter, some wouldn't fit at all. I had a really hard time, given my past adversity to hospital food, reconciling the weight gain. I could remember telling people how great the food was; how good the ice cream, pudding, jello felt sliding coolly down my throat, and those milk shakes--they gave me a lot of those milk shakes, the ones I now termed "Old Lady Shakes", the ones they gave grandma in the nursing home. I could remember also saying once that I'd walk through a swamp full of alligators for one of them. Ensure shakes, 300 calories apiece. I got five a day plus three full meals. No wonder I was no longer the size ten I had maintained for 20 years. Why? Why did they let me eat so much? Must have really been sick to gain weight in the hospital; I must have been sick.

I began to question my family. How come you let them feed me so much? No one really had an answer until I interrogated our middle son, David. "They said you were undernourished and borderline anemic." What?! Undernourished?! I was at the right weight for my height.

"They said you weren't, Mom."

"David, I'm 5'5" if I stretch. 125-130 pounds is plenty."

"Oh, 5'5", Mom?

David, now forever dubbed my "dumb son" happened to be there one day while they weighed me. Instead of just measuring me, error on their part, they asked David how tall I was.

"Well, she's always been taller than me. I'm 5'8", she must be 5'9"."

Having lost a little weight at that point, when you calculate the current weight against a 5'9" frame, it should have been a cause for concern. But even had they given me my heels back (which is what always made me seem much taller to David), the calories wouldn't have distributed on my frame any differently. Twenty pounds--I'd gained 20 pounds because of that miscalculation. I must have been really sick to not notice that before now. Must have been real sick to gain 20 pounds in a hospital. Oh, well, when I got home, I'd get it down, maybe.

Now that everyday awareness was back, I could look around the room at plants, stuffed animals, the grocery bags full of cards and letters, and items hung on the walls. Marilyn, my little Jewish friend, had brought me a copy of "foot prints" that had hung near me even when I couldn't remember. The same verse hung in my office and my home. It had always brought comfort, and she knew it and cared enough to keep it near me for those weeks. On some level, I'm sure it did. There were flowers from the Insurance Women's National Officers. I'd look at them and smile and say to myself, "Well, you didn't kill me. I'm still alive." I had been exhausted when I returned from Denver but had too much to do to rest. I knew I was tired. I had even said to Doug, "Sure would be nice to be just sick enough to go to the hospital for a few days and just rest." Guess it isn't only prayers that can get answered. I'll surely be careful of statements made in the future. I started going through the bags of cards again, rereading them. Women, special women from all over the country, had taken time to send a thought, well wishes, prayers. They would be forever special. I would put these in scrapbooks when I got home. I'd save them always, and I'd be well enough to go to conventions next year.

There had been phone calls before that were lost because of my memory, but the ones that came now added joy to my day. How rich I was, even if I had to give up all the things I'd worked so hard for in the past. I had my family and many friends. Who could want any more? What a joy it was to just be alive. I was becoming more aware of just how close I'd come. Bits and pieces, little

flashes of memory came and stuck. But there were days that would forever be lost in that dark area of fear and confusion where I believe, now more than ever, that I had lived so long saying, "I don't have time to be sick. I always take care of everyone else." My brain was not only confused by the blood, it couldn't reconcile that Sue could be "physically sick", so it rationalized "crazy" instead.
Super-woman could not possibly have been knocked off her feet by something physical.

Super-woman died that September evening of 1990. I had a memorial of her while I was still in the hospital. I might occasionally miss her, but I sure didn't want her back. Someone else could have a turn, and,if they were my friends, I'd encourage them to be sure to give her periodic leaves of absence so they could avoid a real scary, real expensive, trip to Indiana.

Dr. "I want to be God" Thomas was talking to me. They didn't see anything different. There was a blockage in the temple area. They didn't know why, but tiny vessels fingered out from it to carry blood to the frontal lobe. They didn't know why the blood vessels broke--could have always been weak--but he didn't think surgery was recommended now. They would want to do another MRI later, but for now, there was nothing further he could do. He didn't know it then because I didn't say it, but I had no intention of letting anyone cut into my head and, least of all, this doctor, who, in my opinion, had no bedside manner at all. (This was later to change for both of us.) I'm sure he thought then that I was as bad a patient as I thought he was a doctor.

They were now talking about letting me go home. I could do outpatient therapy, and they would see me periodically for medical checks. I was going to finally go home. Doug had been able to take me on short outings away from the hospital that month, but now they were really going to send me home for good. That would be great; the kids could come over. I could have my things, sleep in my bed. We began a discharge plan. Marilyn would do my speech and cognitive therapy. She brought Danny back. I had to have her. I trusted her. Because she was now attached to a local community re-entry program, I'd have the other there also. My daughter-in-law also worked there, so it was not unfamiliar to me. Because they wouldn't let me drive, Doug could drop me off there as he took Danny onto his. Although Danny was driving some, when the weather looked bad, we weren't going to take any chances that first year.

Everything all arranged, I began to pack up my things. Doug and I made our tour to the different floors and wings I had been on to say goodbye to all the nurses, who through their caring, had become special to me. I even had an opportunity to return the favor of a visit to Tony, the giant of a man who had picked me out of bed one night and whose voice saying "I've got you" gave me a safe haven for a few minutes, as it was his turn to be in the hospital bed. Tony had been hit by a car, had two broken knees and was now accepting care instead of giving it. I was sure glad I was not the insurance agent who took the young woman's accident report. It would have been very difficult to maintain a professional air, as well as a straight face, and type "I didn't see him". Tony was mending and so was I. We said goodbye. If I ever get sick again, I hope his is a voice that forms an island of safety in the sea of uncertainty.

I found Kristen and embraced her, thanked the many others, and returned to my rehab bed for the last night. I was elated at going home. They probably were, for want of a better word, relieved to see me leave.

Arms full the next morning, we said our last goodbyes. As we were approaching the lobby, a small blond woman came up and threw her arms around my neck.

"Mom woke up this morning, she knows us. Thank you for talking to us, for being here."

"Thank you, God, for giving me a way to begin turning this awful experience into a good one. Please help me continue to do so," I prayed as we left the sisters. They were on their way up to help their mom start her journey to wellness. I was on my way home!

> You grieve differently from other people--not so differently that you cannot find fellowship in suffering with them, yet so differently that no one else's grief is exactly like your own.
>
> --Wayne E. Oates

> Some patients, though conscious that their condition is perilous, recover their health simply through their contentment with the goodness of the physician.
>
> --Hippocrates

CHAPTER 16

As I left the hospital this time, there was no fear, no anger, just joy. I was alive. I was so blessed. I had all I needed, and over the past years had acquired many of the things I wanted. Life was going to be better than ever. I didn't make promises lightly, and I had promised myself to work to be the best that I could be. I would do that, I <u>could</u> do that. Danny had worked so hard, allowed me to push him, and had made great strides. I could hardly do less. I had cut a Garfield cartoon out a number of years before to show to Danny and to use as a take-off for a piece in the Head Injury Chapter newsletter. Garfield had been on a diet with very little success. When asked what he was going to do about missing his goal, he replied, "I'll lower my expectations." Danny had never lowered his, and I had no intention of being less than what I had demanded from Danny. Not giving in became as much of a struggle as the deficits I now dealt with.

While in the hospital, I got up and dressed, ate, took myself to therapy, and went outside to smoke. At home, I had to do it all on my own. The problem, believe it or not, was compounded because I had no physical deficits. To anyone who has not experienced it, I'm sure that sounds like the most ludicrous statement in the world. Many would feel that I didn't know how lucky I was not to have any. I did know! But when people can't see it, often they also don't believe it. Doug had been there from the onset. He had traveled with me during my out-of-body experiences--so called now because my mind went to Indiana, New York, and various other places, including home to get my van and check myself into the hospital while my body never left the hospital bed.

When I carried some of my belongings through the door, wearing my "Power Suit" and high heels, he saw me as being well, also. He had wanted it so badly for so long, that the wish helped flesh out the thought. I looked well. I talked well. I walked well, but my head, which had kept track of three people's schedules and a myriad of committees, causes, and business items, now couldn't keep track of time, couldn't remember if she took her pills, and could only stay on one track at a time. If I were getting dressed, that's all I could do. There was no more start dinner, throw a load of clothes in, review notes for a meeting coming up, and make sure Doug and Danny were all set. I looked as though I could do it, but I couldn't.

We had, over the years, developed compensatory strategies for Danny. Now, it was time to find some for me. I tried moving the pill bottle from one side of the sink to the other and then couldn't remember which side was which. I turned it upside down, but that could have been from the time before. Sticky notes, God's gift to office personnel--on one side, it said "Take pill", on the other "Took pill". Just the whole process of moving the paper around and plopping the bottle down, created enough physical activity and thought process, to facilitate the automatic transference from short-term to long-term memory, which was still occurring given the eight hours between pills then became manageable. (Short-term memory, that thought process which allows you to recall a phone number dialed five minutes earlier, still evaded me; however, somehow I could dredge up that same phone number eight <u>hours</u> later.)

I couldn't look at a lot of things and make a decision. Too much visual stimulus made my brain reel. I had to learn to look in my closet in segments, to scan almost made me dizzy. Because I couldn't drive, I was now a very tense passenger. I'd never been a good one; now it was worse: (1) because the law wouldn't let me drive and (2) neither would the doctor or Doug. If I looked straight ahead, things going by on the side, particularly when sunlight shining through the trees produced a strobe light effect in my peripheral vision made me feel almost dizzy. The motion of the van, a sway or motion in the rear, set off an alarm somewhere in my balance system that was almost painful in the discomfort it caused. I never had suffered from motion sickness, and some of these new feelings were awful. They didn't just go away, but something new was coming. This was Michigan, and winter was just around the corner bringing ice and snow and bad roads. Now it's one thing to be a gasping passenger on dry roads; on the icy roads, I got verbal.

Marilyn kept telling me my verbal skills were very good. I had that to be thankful for, because if I could talk things through, I could help my memory, make people understand and even to plan my day. She didn't say I should use those same skills to lash out at Doug, rage at the kids and scream into the phone at the insurance company, but I did that, too.

I had, all my life, carried anger at a multitude of things as excess baggage; but it was always closely held, and I could let it loose or rein it in at will. I could be and often was a formidable opponent in an argument and I had honed the skills needed to be a first class "Bitch" over the years; I guess I took pride in how those had been used on several occasions. Dealing with hospitals, physicians, therapists and the insurance company for eight years, fighting for what I perceived as "Danny's life", I had had a lot of practice.

What I found when I came home was there were no longer reins on that anger. One small remark would act like a match thrown on a pile of gasoline-soaked rags and I would explode into this roaring woman who was fighting mad, right now. If conversation continued, the anger escalated as flames would if more gasoline were poured on the fire. I couldn't control it. After this happened three or four times, it began to scare me. My kids had often made fun of me and they played off TV commercials, "When my Mom talks, people listen", "You don't want to make my Mom mad. You won't like it, if you make her mad." Their list went on and on. Not often were they the targets of my anger, but they felt comfortable, I know, in their belief that I'd fight to the death for any of them if they were in the right. Not having a mother who did that, I was determined my children would always have the advocacy that comes with a mother's love. God bless them; they were all normal, healthy kids who were often in difficult situations, and they gave me lots of practice with teachers as well as neighbors. But that was often rehearsed anger, or simmering and slowly-moving-to-boil anger. Now, I was full blown mad right now; and it got worse, not better.

One night, Danny, who was also feeling the stress my illness had put on the family when I had forgot something he'd told me twice before, turned to me and raised his voice on the third explanation, and added a smart comment. I spun around and got right up in the face of this, my almost six-foot, baby and explained not only that I might forget, I might have brain damage, and although he might be a brown belt, I was still his mother, still the boss, and he had better not <u>ever</u> think he was <u>old</u> enough or <u>big</u> enough to challenge me! Our son, David, the dumb one, watched his 5'5" mother (not the 5'9" one) blaze into action, with his mouth open. He told me afterwards he was sure glad I hadn't been like that when he was growing up.

"I've never seen anger in your eyes like that, Mom. I'd never have lived if you'd been like that before. Are you okay?"

I wasn't okay; I had been out of control; and it scared me. I thanked God that night I did not have small children because I might have hurt them if I had

had to put up with the everyday exploits of three-, four-, or five-year-olds. Could I be trusted to have my beloved grandchildren around? What if I couldn't? I loved them so much. I wanted them back, a very real part of my life, but I couldn't risk hurting them. I had to get this under "control". I needed help. I got more therapy--biofeedback techniques, talked with the psychologist and with my Pastor. Never in my life had anything or anyone controlled me, and this anger wasn't going to either. There was still some blood in the frontal lobe, which had helped me rationalize some of the changes early on, and,maybe as it went away, I'd be better. I sure hoped so.

Doug and I were having our share of heated arguments, and now we talked. I tried to tell him how out of control I was, that the anger didn't escalate because I willed it; it just happened. He needed to help me not fight back, and he had to, for my sanity, fight differently. Over the twenty years of our marriage, he won most arguments by using the sports tactic--the "best defense is a good offense". If I were mad, he'd get madder. It worked 9 out of 10 times, and he had used it quite effectively. Now, I couldn't back off. I finally had him convinced I couldn't control it. Would he, for awhile if I were escalating, not give into me, but at least just stop the discussion and please, please not raise his voice above mine so that we leapfrogged to a point where we both might be sorry. Once again, as he had done over and over in the past 20 years, his love for me came before what he felt he needed for himself, and I know he often bit his tongue in the weeks to come.

He was assigned a place on my rehab team. He was to be my home monitor. That sibling tattler all kids hate. He was to report things he saw which he felt were concerns. Well, he reported, and I got angry. He used his own personal yardstick to measure my actions; which in some cases is not necessarily a problem. But when you're married to a left brain, linear thinker, a perfectionist, a person who, if you ask him what time it is, he will tell you how to build a watch, and if you persist on the time, will then give you hour/minute/second, after checking the time zone so he knows he's exact. Believe me, it can cause problems. We had had two glaring examples of that measure before the straw finally broke the camel's back.

The first one was over Christmas letters I had designed to send to our policyholders instead of cards. Cards didn't say what I wanted these wonderful people to know. When I reported later I had sent out 1,500 of them, Doug said no and I argued. He told the team that I was getting off track, that 1,500 wasn't the correct amount. I was furious! He was nitpicking. Okay, so I mailed 1,368 after sorting through labels and picking out double households, but I had drafted, designed, typed the letter, took it to the printer, ordered the address labels and checked them, bought the stamps, and put them in the mail--not a small feat for someone who was near death 90 days before and who couldn't find her way out of a room 60 days before. I could be exact, but 50 years from now, would that 132 make a difference? It would to Doug. I hadn't been correct at 1,500. Not paying attention.

The second happened when we took a trip, a promised getaway, out west. In finding my aunt's new home north of Phoenix, we were watching for exits and following the directions. I'm looking for the exit names when Doug said, "How many miles is it?"

"How would I know?"

"Well, you should know. Figure it out."

"Why do I care? Have you let us run out of gas again?"

"Do I pray for a gas station?" I retorted.

"No, but if you're watching the signs, you should be able to figure the miles."

Made perfect sense to him, he did it all the time. He liked to know miles. I, on the other hand, rarely let my gas gauge fall below a quarter, and it wasn't even of interest ever. I had usually figured distance in time, not miles. I could drive to Cincinnati in less than 5 hours on a good day. It took 20 minutes to get Danny to therapy. I was 11 minutes from the hospital in an emergency. If it weren't an emergency, then it was 20. Time had governed my life for so long, almost everything but sex was governed by the clock, and sometimes that might have been too, when I was coming home late at night from a meeting and the clock said 2:00 and Doug was asleep. He had thought it would be good therapy. I needed to be more observant. He had his reasons.

After we came home, a letter to Doug from the rehab facility came in the mail. I opened it. Inside, sent to him, were progress notes, test scores. I was a grown woman, I had signed the rehab contract, and they were sending my husband, who, by the way, was not my guardian, all these things. Test scores showing grade school equivalents in some areas would only give him further ammunition to keep me from doing things. They were reporting to him. How dare they! I stayed in control that evening--seething inside. The envelope in my purse, I'd handle it tomorrow.

Morning came, I got ready for therapy, and arrived there at nine, envelope in hand, anger mounting, and determination clicking with every heel strike on the cement. The first stop was the rehab director's office. No more, no more mail to Doug. The second was the office of my case manager, whom I had grown to admire because of her very real skills at working with those of us who, on occasion, were one bubble off center. I called her the Paginini of case managers. This day she was also instructed to not give Doug any information on me and to be advised he had been fired off my team. I had just fired him, and they were to tell him nothing. Next stop, Marilyn! Where is Marilyn? She was late that morning. I sat in the lounge, drank coffee and simmered. When she walked in the lounge, which in past weeks I had taken to calling my office, I waved the papers at her.

"These were sent to Doug. He can't see this. He already smothers me. Retest me, retest me now!"

The fight or flight response was full blown again. Adrenaline coursed through my system. Marilyn, being not only my therapist but my friend, knew instinctively that I needed to take action as well as see improvement. We redid the tests. I did much better. Doing the tests soothed the anger, but,as I left therapy and went to my office, I was still simmering. They had reported to my husband as if I were a child.

I sat at my desk surveying the wasteland it had become, angry at the facility, angry because I was smarter than those tests showed, angry because Doug kept such close track of me, and getting angrier because all I could do at that desk was sit and make piles. Then I'd sort through the piles and make more. I'd been doing that for weeks. I could answer insurance questions. Anything I knew before was still there. I could do the forms. I was even getting better at talking to irate policyholders. I had called myself a fireman for years--one of my jobs was to put out fires. Now, with a calmer attitude, I could put them out faster; and each success only reinforced this new-found method of confronting anger. I may have had that to feel good about, but I still made those awful piles. Sitting and staring at those piles, one day I put my head in my hands and said, "Oh, God, you made me Doug." My neat orderly desk consistently looked like the disaster across the hall.

Day after day, I fought the battle of the piles of paper, and I always lost until that day I went raging into therapy and fired Doug from the team. When I sat at my desk that afternoon,I decided the piles had to go, too, and they did. Some of the material was outdated. I threw it away. Others were taken to front office staff and delegated. Some was filed, and others put in newly created folders in a stand-up file. The desk was polished and my office, once again, looked like mine. The "pile gremlin" had been banished forever--never, after that day, to darken my office door. Feeling almost euphoric over my accomplishment, I walked into Doug's office and suggested that if he made me mad a couple more times, I might be cured! (He was not amused.) Danny had offered once to do it for five dollars; I'd be even cheaper than that. He didn't think that was funny, but I did; and I was more determined than ever to keep a sense of humor about everything I could, as well as pull as much back under my control as possible. If I were to be well, I needed to expect I would be well and be satisfied with what I could do at that moment, adding more activities weekly until I was back in full control of my life.

Once the office was clean, it was nicer to sit at my desk and that allowed me to feel more in control. When Doug had Kiwanis or another meeting over the lunch hour, I would get a sandwich and lunch at my desk, often reading through the mail order catalogues which appeared daily. One day, as I sat reading through the second one, it occurred to me I really couldn't remember what I had seen in the first one. As I started to look at it again, the laughter started, and the more I laughed, the harder I laughed. Denise, always on alert, must have thought I'd lost the rest of my mind. As I held the two catalogues, I knew at that point I'd never need anymore. By the time I finished one, the other was brand new again. All I needed was two catalogues to keep me entertained. Or two books, or two tapes. When you can't remember, it doesn't take much. I thought it was hysterical.

Denise was concerned. Laughing at limitations is not always easy, but it certainly was better for me than being worried about it. If it never got better, Doug would be better off financially; I wouldn't remember I wanted to order something either.

When I left the hospital, I had expected to not drive for six months. But my wonderful Dr. Wardner had ordered a driving evaluation three weeks before this upheaval, and I had passed with flying colors. I was even more convinced that I was ready to be back on the road after this outburst, and, when I left the office that day, I grabbed a set of Wayne Dyer tapes that had traveled thousands of miles with me the previous year and put them in their place between the seats. I was coming back, maybe a little at a time, but I was coming back. How we had once rejoiced at even the smallest gain that Danny made--when he could bend his fingers purposefully around an Atari joystick, when he took one faltering step, the weeks, months, and years he'd struggled--and I was having fits over three or four months. "Oh, please, God, ignore this old whiner." I would settle, and I would be thankful. Grateful for the progress of today and work to make a little more tomorrow.

"On The Road Again", a good title for a country song. The independence of steering my own course felt good. I pushed in the first tape and adjusted the car seat. Coffee cup in one hand, had to have that traveler (now, if some automaker ever came up with a vehicle that could have a coffee faucet, they'd get my money), and cigarette in the other, I listened to the familiar tones of Dr. Wayne Dyer. I remembered the tape, knew what was coming next--probably if his talk had been set to music, I could have sung along. As he talked about emotion, the psychology of more, not letting other people control you, it all came back. How I had tried the year before to make sense of what he said and put it into practice while I rode the merry-go-round my life had become, not only riding one horse but jumping on one and then the other while the music played and attempted from each and every horse to grab the brass ring. I would set out to do one thing, and I could do that but only for awhile; then I would lapse back into the known, the familiar. Maybe because it was easier, but most probably because there were too many other things in my memory bank that caused road blocks and detours. I listened; it made sense. I knew now that some of it felt real good when applied and "Yeah, Wayne!" I can do that! And I could, I was, and it felt so good. I knew right then I could start putting those things into practice, and I could do them and keep doing them. I could hear. I could understand. I was like the old saying, "When the pupil is ready, the teacher will appear". I was ready. I was open. I was brand new. Maybe a little brain damaged, but I was new, and I knew I could do those things and keep doing many of them. This started a whole new line of thought.

I could have died on the bathroom floor that night if Doug hadn't been home, but I didn't. Was there a new purpose for my life? Or did I, like Danny, have an opportunity to go back to square one and maybe this time, with no adults in my life, to write the scripts I would replay for years, there to say the wrong things? Was I now the way God had really intended this human being to be? I wondered.

Many books compare the mind to a computer in its ability to store facts, to search memory banks, to recall information stored by sight, sound, taste, smell. There was also the old saying, GI-GO, garbage in-garbage out. When the GI-GO came from my memory bank, I had to smile because from way back, to the time Danny was three and his favorite book was Shel Silverstein's, "Where the Sidewalk Ends", one of his favorite pieces was "Sarah Cynthia Sylvia Stout Would Not Take the Garbage Out." A little girl who could and would do everything and anything but take the garbage out. Maybe that children's verse applies more to an insurance woman in her forties than a child. She wouldn't do it, but I'm not so sure the old programs hadn't been in me so long that I couldn't take them out. But the one split second it had taken that blood vessel to burst and send brain cells running for cover had erased many old tapes, or maybe God just hit the accept key and got rid of the whole program. Could have been a little bit of both; but at that moment, one blink in the eye of eternity, all the frustration, all the anger for my body failing me, even though I denied it, was gone and a new peace took over my being. If it never got any better than this, that was okay. If I had an opportunity to go back to the day it all happened, I would do it all again. If it got me to here, where I sat today with this new feeling, new perspective on life, I'd do it again. There was a way to go yet, but I'd do it again. I believed then as I believe now, "if this is brain damage, I'll take it". It sure beats what I was doing and had been doing to myself for years. Besides I could still laugh; still hug my grandbabies; watch all my children prosper; and see Danny continue to do new and different things, all of which he was never supposed to do after his accident. I did have all I needed. I could live with brain damage. At least, I admitted I had it. Some people were uncomfortable when I admitted it. My daughter, Denise, came running back to my office one day as she heard the following come from my office after I hung up the phone.

"I'm the one with brain damage, I'm the one in therapy every day, I'm the one they are determined to make better than new, and they let those people run around out there and give them jobs so they can drive me crazy."

"Please don't keep saying you have brain damage," were the first words out of her mouth. Concern showed in her eyes.

"I do have brain damage. I'm not ashamed of it. We know there are many things I can do, but you more than anyone except maybe Dad know there's so many things that are still hard. Denise, I have brain damage." I walked around the desk and hugged her, hoping to smooth the wrinkles of concern. I'm sure it's an uncomfortable phrase to many people because they see it as a population set apart, but I'm not sure that many of us come through the bike accidents, playground mishaps, skating spills of childhood, or blows from sports, without some. We just haven't had it diagnosed. I chose to keep it out in the open, rather than hide it away like the old crazy aunt in an attic. The garbage had been taken out, and I was not going to gift wrap this and start a new store room. I would not take out ads in the paper with "You, Too, Could Have·Brain Damage", "Brain Light", or "Brain Damage, Don't Leave Home Without It" under my picture. But I was also not about to let it consume me or let it be me, like I had seen happen, not only to the injured and their families, but like we've all seen when a disease, cancer, has invaded a part of the body but the mind of that person as well. Besides, what I had left of my mind, I had other plans for. There's an old Russian saying, "If you are a hammer, all the world looks like a nail". I'd been that hammer for years before the aneurysm. Now, I wanted to be just as purposeful as a hammer's blow but much softer, more touchable, more real. "Yeah, Wayne!" I can do that. Even with brain damage.

I then shall live as one who's been forgiven,
I'll walk with joy to know my debts are paid;
I know my name is clear before my father,
I am his child and I am not afraid.
So greatly pardoned, I'll forgive my brother;
The law of love I gladly will obey.

I then shall live as one who's learned compassion,
I've been so loved that I'll risk loving too;
I'll know how fear builds walls instead of bridges
I'll dare to see another's point of view.
And when relationships demand commitment,
Then I'll be there to care and follow through.

Your kingdom come around and through and in me,
Your power and glory, let them shine through me;
Your hallowed name O may I bear the honor and may
Your living kingdom come in me.
The bread of life O may I share with honor,
And may you feed a hungry world through me.

--Copyright 1980 by William Gaither

> Perseverance is more prevailing than violence, and many things which cannot be overcome when they are together, yield themselves up when taken little by little.
>
> --Plutarch

CHAPTER 17

Denise wasn't the only one who was uncomfortable. The end of January was to be a reunion of the Black Sheep Squadron, five of us from the 1989-90 National Board, in San Antonio, Texas. Doug and I had a condo available to us there at no cost. It had been arranged before I had gotten ill. Tickets sat, paid for, at the travel agency while I laid in the hospital traveling around the country for free. When doctor and therapist felt it was okay for me to fly, Doug, with only a little reluctance, agreed to let me go. There would be others with me all the time, and my pseudo-daughter, Linda, who had been one of our staff and my right arm in Insurance Women before a new job for her husband transferred them to San Antonio, would meet me at the airport, stay with me until my Sheep friends arrived, and then would come back to see I was not alone 'til I was on the plane home. Linda also was the mother of a little blonde imp named Jenna, who called me Nana, and Doug was sure they would watch over me.

I was to have my first go at real independence. Just the thought of it was exhilarating. I felt like a teenager about to go on the Senior Trip. Purse slung over my shoulder, I kissed Doug goodbye and boarded the plane. I had booked a window seat months before because I had always preferred them, but, as I set my purse down next to the cabin wall and fastened the seat belt, I wondered if I had erred in not trying to change that. What if that motion thing I now felt in my head caused me to be sick? Wouldn't I be better off to have an aisle seat? Well, too late now. Turn the air on, put your head back and relax, breathe evenly, in through your nose, out of your mouth. Stay relaxed and see what happens. We were going down the runway. Was I doing the right thing? Could I do this? What if I missed the connection from Dallas to San Antonio? What if I couldn't find my way around?

My self-confidence had been dealt a horrid blow from the big bang of 1990, and, although I talked a good show, I wasn't sure I could perform now I was at center stage. But I also knew that in the same way I had pushed Danny more than once out of his comfort zone, I had to push myself out of mine. I certainly had pushed Danny--"You can do it", "Don't tell me you're tired", "We'll slack off this summer"--all my own words danced around like Marley's ghost in my head. Even Danny had said when I came home from the hospital, "Remember how you pushed me, Mom? I'm going to be on your butt all the time." That comment was much easier to take from him than the night he said, "You know, Mom, maybe God let me have a head injury so I could help you." That night I cried as I held him and assured him that people have accidents; God doesn't cause them, but he's there to get us through. I also thanked God for getting me through all the crises of the past and told him how thankful I was that if my body had to give out, it had been after the time Danny had needed all my strength. Had it been the other way around, I couldn't have pushed him nearly as hard. I knew how tiring just thinking was now, what concentration it took to do things right, and doing something over and over until it was right was not only mentally but physically draining. I'd sure let him play hooky from school more often if it were now. We'd cut back his therapy schedule, too. There were days I'd have taken a beating to be allowed to stay home now, but I knew I had to keep going, and I couldn't let Danny see me expect less of myself than I had of him. He kept me giving 100% just by his presence, this son of mine, a gift from the angels. Surely, he was. How many times did I need that proved to me.

The air was clear, the flight smooth so far. I'd get a pen out of my purse and make some notes for the meeting in Dallas. My purse, where's my purse? I brought the little round black one. I set it on the floor next to the cabin wall, didn't I? Where is it? Questions, concerns, my tickets, money, charge cards were in it. Where was it? Don't panic, you put it right there on the floor. Well, didn't you? I used to joke about liking to talk to myself because sometimes it was the most intelligent conversation I had all day. Now, I was talking to this person with brain damage, who had a memory problem, as well as several others, and, now, I'd lost my purse. Wonderful, just wonderful! I felt around with my heel. There was a bar on the seat; but next to the cabin wall my foot went back, there was a space there. Wait! The purse was narrow. I signalled for the stewardess.

"Excuse me, would you go back about three seats and see if there's a black, round purse next to the cabin wall on the floor?" She just looked at me. "Please?"

Back three seats on the floor, she rescued my runaway purse. "This it?" It sure was. The thrust as we took off and climbed to our current altitude had caused it to slide backward on the uncarpeted area. And I'd figured it out, maybe by accident, but I had my purse in my hand--my money, tickets, credit cards, all there--and my self-confidence had received its first gold star.

I got off at Dallas, had coffee and, of course, replenished the nicotine in my system, found the gate and was on my way to San Antonio. Got another star. Linda met me in San Antonio, and I arranged for a rental car, and we caught each other up to date. The others arrived, we left the airport and I found the condo. Another star! We had a wonderful visit, which lasted four days. Jan (whose husband had died at the same time I went into the hospital) and I commiserated with each other. Gerry and Shari filled us in on their lives, and we all laughed. It felt so good to just laugh, to be away from all the things that reminded me of illness. Here I could be well, no one babied me or treated me any different than they had before. I needed that.

Our good time was only a little dampened by a business meeting we had to drive to Dallas for; but even though it did take away from our time together, it did wonders for my belief that I really had given to and been a part of an association of caring women. Women from all over the United States, many of whom had sent cards to me that filled grocery bag after grocery bag in my hospital room--letters, pictures, banners--were now all around me, asking how I was, saying how well I looked, and arms around me. How special these women were. How fortunate I was to be a part of this insurance sisterhood. How fortunate to be able to be here.

Vacation over, it was time to go home. I was back at the airport. Jenna and I played peek-a-boo around the columns on the concourse. We laughed. We were enjoying life as some older women who observed our play "sniffed" the air. Too bad they hadn't learned to appreciate the sheer joy in the laugh of a child or had their heart touched by "Here I am, Nana." How unfortunate for them.

I had dropped everyone off at the terminal, determined to take the rental car back by myself. Everything was to be a test; they made me do them in therapy; I could make up my own in real life. Went without a hitch--I got another stripe. I might be a full-blown colonel soon. As I sat with Linda, waiting to board for Dallas, I felt the best about me that I'd felt for weeks. Doug's allowing me to do this had been an important growth step. I needed desperately to know that if something happened to him I could do things on my own and not be scared to step off into the unknown, secure in the knowledge I was capable of getting through it. Must remember that Danny may be feeling that way also, can't not let him try, if that's what he wants, even if he's scared to.

When I first came home, I had been, although not physically, emotionally dependent on Doug. I didn't want him to give up any of his activities. So when he'd leave with Danny for Choi Kwang Do, I'd kiss them goodbye, promise to rest, and within forty-five minutes, I'd be connected to someone by telephone. I was scared to be alone. The doctor had done tests, sent me home, but it could happen again. I could have died if I had been home alone. What if? What if? At least, if I were talking to someone and if something happened, he could send help. Now, here I was 1,500 miles from home, people all around, but about to get back on an airplane where medical help would not be available, and I wasn't afraid. I had built a bridge across that chasm of fear I'd seen parents fight while we worked with the head injury group. Now, I'd experienced it from the other side. As I kissed Linda and then Jenna, feeling her tiny warm arms around my neck, I knew the struggle wasn't over. But just as the plane would go down that runway, take off and climb to its cruising altitude, I had gone down life's runway, and I was climbing. Maybe I'd soar with the eagles, too.

My purse beside me in the seat this time, I lay my head back, preparing for take off and replaying the past week on my personal VCR. How much we had laughed. Lots of internal jogging. It had felt so good. Wasn't even too bad when they made me go to bed one night--turned the TV off on me and threatened to tell Doug. They were my friends; they cared; and their company provided a medicine that no amount of money could have bought. Gerry had gotten upset with me referring to the big bang of 1990, touching my right temple and saying "brain damage", being of the opinion that if you said it, you'd be it. She was concerned that it would hamper progress, and there was, at that time, no way to change her mind. I couldn't convince her that it was my way to validate to myself the screw-ups. It gave me license to forget things, to make mistakes. I didn't call myself stupid or dumb; I just said, "Oh, brain damage." Then I'd set about redoing or rethinking the situation and do it right. The woman who stole my things had followed me to Texas, and I laughingly carried on about her. Gerry wasn't sure that was funny either. Doug hadn't thought it was when I first created her. I had been standing in my closet, a hodgepodge of summer, winter and all-season clothes, not now the organized one I had maintained for years, and couldn't find a sweater I knew I owned. I'd been over and over the hangers, was getting frustrated, and knowing I had to lighten this situation. I went into the bathroom where Doug was shaving and sat upon the counter.

"You know, I know I was in the hospital for a long time. I know you are still a very virile man. I also know you'd be too cheap to pay for sex. But did you have to give her my clothes?"

Doug stopped in mid-stroke and looked at me dumbfounded. The look on his face served to start the laughter. He was not amused. At first, he had thought I might be serious.

"How could you think that? I was at the hospital all the time. I was so scared I'd lose you. There is nothing funny about any of this. And I did not have some other woman over here."

Boy, had I stepped on a hornet's nest, and I wasn't sure I had enough words to slap away the hornets. But I did, and we ended up laughing, holding each other. I needed to laugh, to use humor as a sword against the frustration, and Doug needed me well. We would love and laugh, and someday it would be okay again.

Well, this closet creation flew with me to San Antonio and misplaced a number of things. She was to go to Phoenix with me, also. As a matter of fact, she traveled with me for many miles. But right now we were circling Detroit Metro, waiting to land. Doug would meet me at the gate. I had missed him this trip, really missed him. The first time in a long time. It felt good. Felt like that feeling you experience when you're digging through a drawer and find something you had long ago resigned yourself to the fact it would be gone forever, and then all of a sudden it was there. Felt good.

I came off the plane with half a dozen gold stripes on my arm. I was now on my way to becoming an admiral on the sea of self-confidence. I could drive. I could plan a trip and go out of town by myself. I no longer made piles in the office, and I was ready to take on some of the past responsibilities that I had dumped on so many people unexpectedly when I fell ill. I might even be ready to start reading books again and maybe take another class. Going to Texas had been not only more fun but more productive than my trip to Indiana.

It's good to be just plain happy; it's a little better to know that you're happy and to know why and how and still be happy, be happy in the being and the knowing, well that is beyond happiness, that is bliss.

--Henry Miller

Humor is a prelude to faith
and
Laughter is the beginning of prayer.

--Reinhold Niebuhr

CHAPTER 18

Therapy had been an experience right from the beginning. Marilyn, I'm sure, agreed to be my speech therapist because she was my friend, but the O.T. and P.T. had me because it was their job. I'm not sure I would have wanted me. My daughter-in-law worked there, so they were treating a family member. But I'd been around this business for eight years, was familiar with a great deal of the technical jargon, as well as the treatments, and I had already created a reputation at the hospital and in post- acute-care therapy. I'm not sure I would have wanted to accept me, but they did.

I went to P.T. because of neck pain. My P.T. Stu and I, finally through talk, treatment and paying attention (my staying in tune with me) located the difficulty. When I was intent on a task, concentrating so hard to get it all right, I'd clench my teeth. I found if I stuck a pencil in my mouth, I wouldn't bite down on the back teeth and, therefore, not tighten those muscles, which resulted in neck pain. Since I didn't get lost anymore, P.T. was over.

Now, occupational therapy was different. We'd mastered meal planning, cooking, baking, and banking. Marilyn ran interference for me on the banking. They had me doing deposit slips and account registers, and I'd never liked that nor cared, so we went on to the next step, distractibility. Now, it was time to make sure that I could really do my job at the office. When we had been doing all the housewife things, that was a little depressing. Seemed to me you ought to be able to choose what you forgot. I hated housework and really hated ironing, but I could do it.

Shelly came to work with me. We went out on a physical inspection of an office building to prepare a quote. I passed. My verbal skills were good, and I could now arrange things in their proper order. Numbers still were not my best friends. I transposed them, forgot them, so an adding machine with a tape to doublecheck and recheck now became my new toy and best friend on the desk.

I was not taking over the bills again for real. I'd tried before, wrote the checks but wasn't really sure where we were until now. Finally, we were all paid up on all of them; and I sent letters to all our creditors expressing our gratitude that they had chosen not to turn us over for collection when things had not been paid as in the past. Doug hadn't been concerned and some had not been paid on in months. I'm sure our past credit history helped a lot, but we had many who were very understanding. Made me see creditors in a new light.

Next thing to tackle was the mounting bills for therapy and tests and carryovers from when I was an in-patient. That became a different story. With Danny, we dealt with coverage under the Michigan Auto No-Fault. All bills for the rest of his life for medical care, because of that accident, were to be paid. It was only a matter of securing a doctor's order, and the insurance company was mandated by law to pay the bill. Not so with hospitalization. They pay for coverages listed in the policy, and we had a high deductible with 80-20 co-pay. Some challenge for a person who numbers were not her best friend. Of course, company claims people can also be a challenge, as well as the maze of medical bills you can have for any one medical procedure. A test done in a hospital results in a bill from the hospital, a bill from the technician, a bill from someone who interpreted the test, and the doctor who ordered it and then saw you to explain the results. Insurance companies who are under new cost containment guidelines only exacerbate the situation. The driving evaluation ordered by my doctor cost $100.00. I sent it to the insurance company. They denied payment. I called. They denied payment. I sent a letter to the company president. Still no payment. I sent my therapy bills in--some were paid; the biofeedback was paid under the mental illness coverage of $40.00 per visit, not the therapy amount. Mental illness, mental illness! I wasn't crazy. I had had an aneurysm, a stroke, a bleed. I wasn't nuts. Or was I? I put in a call to Dr. Wardner.

"Am I okay? Am I nuts?"

"No, Sue, you're not. I'll write them a letter. I'll explain."

This was the company I had sold for. Now they were embarrassing me by not knowing what treatments were considered appropriate. They should know it. Shouldn't they? Then another note via payment statement. Therapy treatment, if continued, may be considered maintenance and not eligible for coverage. Once again, I walked around my office, sounding like a small child testing a swear word. Maintenance, maintenance, maintenance! I got nowhere with my claims representative. Once again, I placed a call to my wonderful doctor, who always heard me.

"Maintenance, they are referring to my therapy as maintenance. I've been around this long enough. I understand that maintenance is what they do to keep you mobil or just thinking. Why are they saying this to me? Aren't I improving? Why can't they just pay these bills and quit doing this?"

"Sue, just relax " was the calm, reassuring response of this man I had learned to respect so much, not only for his medical, but his people skills. Of course, putting him on a scale with my neurosurgeon, there was no balance at all. This one talked to me like I was a real person.

"Sue, they aren't connecting your age with the medical problem. They see stroke; they think older patient. Maintenance would apply there."

"Every time I have to send in one of their forms with a stack of bills, it's real clear I'm only 47. Can't they read?"

"Relax, I'll send them a letter. It will be okay."

Once again, I could not believe that our home office would have claims examiners who would do this. But faced with the facts, I had to believe it. I'd write the president of the company. For all I got from that, I could have saved time, paper, and postage. Well, maybe, if I ever got sick again, it would be simpler and easier to just die. That thought did linger but not for long. Would serve them right to have to put up with me again. Maybe my temper would be even worse next time. Maybe I'd even get a lawyer. That certainly would be interesting. Between the hospital billing systems, the insurance companies fortunate to have a hospitalization policy, sometimes getting well is only half the battle. Handling the paperwork can be a challenge for the best of minds, and it was definitely one for me.

Along with my hospital bills, which were now past one hundred thousand, the company was trying to make changes in Danny's recovery program. Just what I needed. Marilyn said it was what I needed, would be good therapy for me. Call a team meeting, meet with the claims people. I'd handled it for years, why not now? Well, maybe not now because I would say or do something that was inappropriate, or not in Danny's best interest. I didn't want to jeopardize one step in his progress. We had come so far. I didn't want to be like the repairman who, while he was on top of a building, kept losing presence of mind. I smiled as I remembered the story but was afraid, given my confidence level, I would do just that.

Most insurance offices abound with photocopies of accident explanations and/or cartoons that spread seemingly like wildfire from one office to the other. Several years before, I had one that had purported to be the explanation of a Worker's Compensation claim, and it read:

Dear Sirs:

I am writing in response to your request for additional information. In block number 3 of the accident report, I put 'trying to do the job alone' as the cause of my accident. You said, in your letter, that I should explain more fully, and I trust that the following details will be sufficient.

I am a sprinkler filter by trade. On the day of the accident, I was working alone on the roof of a new six-story building. When I completed my work, I discovered that I had about 500 pounds of material left over. Rather than carry the material down by hand, I decided to lower it in a barrel by using a pulley which, fortunately, was attached to the side of the building at the 6th floor.

Securing the rope at ground level, I went up to the roof, swung the barrel out and loaded the material into it. Then, I went back to the ground and untied the rope, holding it tightly to insure a slow descent of the 500 pounds of material. You will note in block 11 of the accident reporting form that I weigh 135 pounds. Due to my surprise of being jerked off the ground so suddenly, I lost presence of mind and forgot to let go of the rope. Needless to say, I proceeded at a rather rapid rate up the side of the building. In the vicinity of the third floor, I met the barrel coming down. This explains the fractured skull and broken collarbone.

Slowed only slightly, I continued my rapid ascent, not stopping until the fingers of my right hand were two knuckles deep into the pulley. Fortunately, by that time, I regained presence of mind and was able to hold tightly to the rope in spite of my pain.

At approximately the same time, however, the barrel of material hit the ground, and the bottom fell out of the barrel. Devoid of the weight of the material, the barrel now weighed about 50 pounds. I refer you again to my weight in block number 11. As you might imagine, I began a rapid descent down the side of the building.

In the vicinity of the third floor, I met the barrel coming up. This accounts for the two fractured ankles and the lacerations of my legs and lower body. The encounter with the barrel slowed me enough to lessen my injuries when I fell into the pile of material and, fortunately, only three vertebrae were cracked.

I am sorry to report, however, that as I lay there on the material . . . in pain, unable to stand and watching the empty barrel six stories above me, I again lost presence of mind. I let go of the rope.

The supposed Worker's Compensation claim is a little far fetched, but there are probably insurance people who would say, "No, I've got a better one than that in real life." But often people, unlike our repairman, fail to be accountable for their problems. They would prefer to pass the blame onto someone else. In this case, it was the boss' fault for leaving him alone. I did not want to take the chance, even remotely, that I would be at fault in any way for changing Danny's progress in therapy, but . . . "Marilyn said". I was to take charge of my life and Danny's again. I had to think about it, and for two days, that's about all I did.

Things happen to all of us caused by external as well as internal forces. Mostly, our lives are directed by external forces, beginning with the weather, job layoffs, laws, taxes, and accidents--things we have no control over. External forces often control our lives in ways that we would prefer they didn't--head injury. But how we handle them, our perspective, has to come from an internal force that we can control and sometimes alter the final outcome. I knew that I had to, for Danny's sake, get control of that inner perspective again. I had to pay attention, stay on track, take notes and not for one minute in that rehab meeting could I lose presence of mind.

I sent out letters. I made my notes, researching all past therapies and actions Doug and I had taken. For years, when Doug and I played cards, he had a saying, "Never go to war with a pop gun". I had a file folder that I thought was comparable to a Sherman tank. Marilyn was at the meeting because she still was, after eight years, a very integral part of Danny's team and of his life. She was also there as my speech and cognitive therapist to monitor me. I began tentatively, unsure, not confident I was on very solid ground. Then more neuro-psyche testing was requested, and I couldn't believe my ears. We had had one less than a year before, and they wanted another? I got mad. Marilyn said I had been wandering a little prior to that, almost like falling into the holes in swiss cheese, but she said the minute that I got angry, it all worked. I was on track--clear, concise, exacting, and in control. We went to war; we got what Danny's team thought he needed. I'd made it through, somehow some inner resource came to the surface.

Anger again, the coursing of adrenaline through my body, made it all work. I knew then that this was something else I needed to think about. If I could function when that response of fight or flight kicked in, what was my body telling me? I knew that anger was detrimental to the body. Rages caused heart problems; continuous anger could kill you. Wasn't one of the body chemicals produced during anger adrenalin? If I were so determined to laugh and produce the endorphins that kept you well, was this putting the body into the fight response counterproductive? And when I really thought about it, I had been kicking that response in at will for years. An attorney friend of mine had always called me a "causist"--fight for a cause, raise money for a cause, argue for Danny, sometimes argue for its own sake, push myself into deadline situations, 24th hour preparations, overbook myself so I was always, always functioning under the pressure of the clock, running away from reality, the pain of Danny's injury, the loss he had suffered. Had I done it so long my body, my brain, what was left, was addicted to that chemical rush that gives tiny women the strength to lift automobiles? Was my body addicted to adrenalin like others were to street drugs? I'm not sure even now. My Pastor, who has a psychology/counseling background, thought it might be possible, but we had no evidence. I went in search of some and have been able to draw some of my own conclusions but certainly not based on medical fact.

The words coming from the claims supervisor at this meeting for Danny was not, in my opinion, based on medical fact either. This team meeting regarding Danny's therapy plan only exacerbated my growing anger and outrage at the way our claim on Danny, as well as my own, were being handled. Their feeling was that since Danny was now eight years past injury, there should be a real cutback in therapy. I'm sure they would have preferred none. I heard eight years. How well I understood eight years. I'd been there as well, but I couldn't then nor can I now understand how that was relevant to the case in point.

Given the fact that Danny was within weeks of being ten when his therapy began, those eight years brought many changes for him and would have without a head injury. Puberty changed him physically, as well as emotionally. High school, then graduation, driving, the beginning of college courses, all part of life's landmarks for all of us, where we experience physical and psychological changes, are much more important to deal with properly when the deficits are apparent to the one involved. As parents, we had to handle things differently than with the previous five, and we needed guidance. We had to make sure Danny had all the necessary support systems, and, as always in medicine, time brings changes in techniques, treatment and ideology. There was always the chance we would hit on something that would move Danny closer to complete wellness. Danny might, at any given time, be ready for the "teacher to appear", and I had always wanted him to have the opportunity to be in the right place. How could an adjustor or claims supervisor, who hadn't been there every day, determine anything by timeframe only? Now that Danny has reached nineteen and considered an adult, and now that the biological changes are out of the way, we can start looking at time frames. But I thought then, and still do, that it was an inappropriate reference given the rapid natural changes in the pediatric patient. In fact, there has been documented improvement in adults ten years post injury. In light of that, maybe absurd is a better word.

I had had to argue over my own hospitalization claim for the biofeedback, the driving evaluation, the reference to maintenance, delays in payment, double billings and collection agencies because of it. Now, it appeared that I was dealing with people who had graduated from the College of "Loonie Logic". If you've not heard of that particular school of thought, let me explain "Loonie Logic".

If given the question, "Why are fire trucks painted red?", our group of virtual brain trusts would deduce the following:

There is 12" to a foot.

A foot is a ruler.

Queen Elizabeth is a ruler.

Queen Elizabeth is the name of a ship.

Ships sail on the oceans.

There are fish in the ocean.

Fish have fins.

Fins hate Russians.

Russians are red.

Firetrucks are always rushin', so "We'll paint them red."

Eight years of therapy--zap! You're cured. Given your age, maintenance. We're not going to continue to pay. Biofeedback, we only pay a portion on mental illness. "Loonie Logic"? Could be. How appropriate the cartoons that talk about the major cause of stress coming from dealing with insurance policies.

It also became very apparent that it was once again time to make a doctor change for Danny. We needed a doctor with a fresh perspective. One who could view him and his problems as a young adult, and just exactly as they were, not one who had seen improvement but was looking with the insurance company at a calendar. Also, we wanted one who would not be so wrapped up in his own hospital-based program that it would serve as blinders with regard to what else might be available. Also, we needed one we could feel would place long-term patient benefit ahead of insurance company current dollar.

I used to really try and sell insurance. I would talk about today's dollar and future dollars. You will probably buy more with today's dollars than those of tomorrow. It seems to me that it makes more sense to invest in strong rehab programs which may make a change for the better now, than wait and pay more later. Makes sense to this insurance person, but claims are paid on policies already sold, and sometimes it takes a better man than the cartoon character "Charlie Brown"; sometimes it takes a Mom to meet the challenge.

When I was in the early stages of recovery, Doug said he tried to get the doctors to say stress caused the bleed. He wanted to have his heavy artillery when we fought the war of "Now, you're going to slow down". Best he could get was a maybe but also "That it may have brought it on early", but it would have happened eventually anyway given the configuration of the blood vessels. Well, he didn't have a Sherman tank, but he certainly had more than a pop gun. He also had a wife who had wrestled with insomnia for years, who now was asleep the minute her head hit the pillow. One who now could fall asleep in a chair in front of the TV, who slept one day for an hour and a half head down at the kitchen table. Certainly had a real power house to hold back. Someone just chomping at the bit to get back into a harness. The fact that I wasn't was a joy to Doug and an ever growing concern for me. When is the passion coming back? When?

This I Believe

I believe that life is for living
for rising in the morning with
a smile on my face
from the simple joy of being me
and being alive.
I believe that my success in this day
will depend on my outlook,
my openness and my optimism.
I believe that this day
offers possibilities
to change for the better,
and opportunities
to reach for the best.
I believe that real happiness
is all around me, and that
it is as near as the
voice of a friend
the whisper of my love,
and the thought of my family.
I believe that eyes
are made for beholding
arms are made for enfolding
and hearts are meant to say . . .
That for all its wrongs and worries,
my life is right for me,
and thanks to my efforts,
it will only get better
this I truly believe.

--Douglas Richards

CHAPTER 19

While Doug and I were driving through the southwest on our "Let's get away from sickness" vacation, we saw many once-occupied houses now lying in various stages of disrepair, some no more than a few stones that once were a wall or the shell of a fireplace.

One day I said to him, "How sad, that was once somebody's dream." His blank look and my explanation took a little away from my thought, but I reflected on it for days. Someone or some family had moved to that spot once with all their belongings and a dream--to ranch, to farm, to marry, to have children, to have a life, or a better life. Had not Doug and I had a dream when we held Danny for the first time, only minutes old, in the delivery room? Had we not watched that dream grow, develop into a skinny, long-legged, young boy, and then watch over him as that dream was dashed by an accident? Had we not for years been trying to help him rebuild his dream?

Had I not had a dream, plans, goals that had been now replaced by sticky notes, planner pads, second guessing myself, struggles to control anger, no energy, and a loss of the passion that drove me? He didn't make the connection then, maybe he never will. Maybe it would reopen old wounds, hurt too much.

In workshops on death and the grieving process, we learn there are many steps to that process, such as denial, anger, etc.; and that during the recovery process, we must pass through, live each one, confront it, deal with it and move on. In that process comes a healing to our hearts, mind and soul. With a head injury, I wasn't sure with Danny, and I find myself even less sure with me, that the grieving for the people we once were, or could have been, will ever fully be over. For me, it's much simpler because of age. There were so many things already experienced, and I have no physical limitations. But for my son, who makes each one of my days a more treasured item, will he ever quit mourning the loss of baseball or sports in general? Maybe as he grows in other areas, some of it will be replaced by more adult visions and different goals.

Danny's martial arts instructor is on the phone. Since Danny is the first handicapped, closed-head injury victim to achieve the level of black belt, would we consider taking him to the National Headquarters of Choi Kwang Do in Atlanta to let him be part of the first promotional video? Would we consider? This was an opportunity for Danny to receive some positive strokes for all the years of struggle. He would be there if we had to borrow money. It would be a growth experience for Danny, and we could add a couple of days and see our oldest son,

Doug, who lived in Atlanta; an added bonus, I could hug our youngest grandson as well. We made all the arrangements.

Being part of the production of a commercial video is an experience. We went to give Danny an opportunity to receive the "atta boys" we all need to keep going. He went into it with the same attitude that he approached everything.

"I'm nobody special, Mom."

I thought he was special and still admire that inner quality that keeps him going. The cameras moved around on dollies, and Danny did a walk-through. This young man, his competitive spirit locked inside a body that wouldn't cooperate, was handling himself well. I had written an article regarding this special martial arts class for a Michigan Head Injury Alliance booklet years before. In the article, I referred to lilies. Here was Danny, going through the paces, a lily in full bloom.

Lilies of the Field

> Webster defines a lily as pure, white, pale or delicate. The human body, while in a coma, is in a very pure, pale and delicate state. Often life hangs in a very delicate balance. Brain cells die; limbs deteriorate, and the loss is really unknown. The brain, much like the bulb from which the lily grows, spends a time dormant; and then, as the patient emerges from the coma, he is often much different from the person he remembers, skills lost, friends gone, and confronted by an unfriendly world. Through much care and nurturing, such as that given the delicate lily, new beginnings start the process which gives the human flower a purpose.
>
> Sometimes that care and nurturing deviates from the traditional, as in the karate program at the Saline Head Injury Program in Saline, Michigan. In 1986, the program was developed by Kathleen Ponza, physical therapist, and Phillip Kwiencinski,

instructor for the Saline Choi Kwang Do club. They began with a six-week trial period and have now passed the two-year mark. Originally, there were four patients and two aides in the class. During the past two years, the size has changed based on those entering and leaving the program. Only two of the original class members remain. Mike Keller and Danny Hoppe have, after many hours of study and practice, now become red belts and will be testing soon for their next one.

The past two years this martial arts program has taught much more than self-defense. It has given back to Mike and Danny self-confidence and self-esteem. Limbs that previously were, for all practical purposes, nonfunctional, now with the desire to make them move, soon had limited movement with a purpose. Minds that could not remember yesterday retained class terminology and techniques. This was found to carry over into other areas of their therapy and daily lives as well. Inappropriate behavior is often one of the most noticeable consequences of head injury. The courtesy and respect they were required to give their instructor during class time also moved into the therapy sessions and soon went home with them.

In a program adapted and designed to allow them successes with each test, each new belt, the encouragement of their instructor and family members, as well as the special attention and the support of Master Kwang Jo Choi, their enthusiasm and new self-esteem helped them to take another step forward.

Each step after a head injury is into the unknown. They must accept the challenge life has given them--master it, meet their goals, and start the process all over again. One second in time, a blow to the brain robbed them of the person they once were. Much like the lily that blooms and lay dormant again for Mike and Danny, Choi Kwang Do has helped the blossoming of these individuals. As the lily in bloom sways with the breeze, Choi Kwang Do allows them to begin each day with a little more flexibility and tolerance for a world that is just now beginning to understand them.

Danny's Mom

Danny was to be the flower that blossomed, not me. And when they decided that I should be interviewed on camera, I searched my vocabulary for every word I could think of to help get me out of it. I even resorted to the "brain damage" ploy. "I can't do it. I won't be able to remember lines," "Hire someone else; say it's me." There was no way out of this.

For Danny, as always, I'd try. For Danny, I'd fought doctors, therapists, psychologists, teachers, insurance adjustors, hospital administrators for broader programs. For Danny, I'd gladly give my life. For Danny, I could talk to a video camera, and maybe I could help encourage others like Danny to take the challenge of "Pil Sung" (certain victory) over what some might think were limitations. We are often only bound by limitations we think we have. It becomes the self-fulfilling prophesy over and over again. Danny never bought into that philosophy. He was, once again, leading me, teaching me, forcing me, for him, to walk outside my comfort zone so I could grow a little more. It was good for Danny, and this time it was also good for me. It was another test to see if I still had the mettle to stand and stare in the face of something I feared and stare it down. I could. I did.

We made the video, and it's now out there on the international market for everyone to see. How far a determined little boy can come when given a chance. Danny made the papers and did a local TV show. I was the mother of a star. Well, I told everybody I was. Achieving the level of black belt is no small feat for someone without physical limitations and memory deficits, but the desire to achieve has to be stronger than the feeling of "I'll never make it". "I could never do that". "I'll look funny", or the variety of negative responses we can feed ourselves instead of the mentally nutritious, positive responses.

John C. Maxwell, in his book, Your Attitude/Key to Success, writes about "flat world thinking". I like that phrase better than negative because I think it says it all. He writes about flat world statements and then suggests ways to make the world round. When trauma strikes, we are often knocked flat, or like a tire with the air gone we become flat. In that condition, if we allow it, we can develop attitudes that mimic the way we think and feel. If we allow them to continue, if we don't change thought processes and vocabulary, our actions into positive, purposeful, forcing forward momentum, we stay flat. Not every family has a Danny, but every family has within it the resources to become the tire pump, when the tire needs air.

Lord, make me an instrument of Your peace.
Where there is hatred, let me sow love;
where there is injury, pardon;
where there is doubt, faith;
where there is despair, hope;
where there is darkness, light;
and where there is sadness, joy.

--St. Francis of Assisi

CHAPTER 20

The video was an experience, but life and therapy were reality, and it awaited our return to Michigan. We were cutting back on my therapies, and I was spending more time in the office, trying to pull the pieces back together. My organizational skills were so-so. If I did it before, I could do it now from memory. If you gave me something new to pull together, it took hours. Some of the time was spent in checking and rechecking. My self-confidence was so low, I still could not trust myself to do it right the first time. But the same determination that once had driven Danny was held out before me, written on the blackboard of memory--don't quit, keep struggling, be persistent in your efforts to get it right and build on that foundation as a frame of reference for the successes of tomorrow. Danny continued to teach me by the example he had set so many years before. Much like the Chinese who have no word that translates to our word "problem"; neither did Danny; neither would I.

I was at a point where if I were well enough to go to the office, I should be well enough to get back into the swing of things as far as meetings were concerned--church, Insurance Women.

One of the program speakers at an Insurance Women's meeting spoke on stress and the mind's reaction to it. Her example of how P.O.W.'s used their brains to preserve their minds during their confinement was intriguing. Had I been so afraid of death, so out of control, that my mind wrote its own script for self-preservation? Interesting. I was still bent on finding out about how my liking for the adrenalin rushes might have provoked the bleed but also I needed some more information on using humor as not only a wellness tool, but I wanted other validation to those around me that the emergency room humor I had developed wasn't sick, wasn't preemptive of a worsening of attitude, and it was okay.

She gave me the name of C. W. McCabe in Colorado, who had a tape series, "Humor Risk and Change". I ordered it, and he gave me all the ammunition I needed to convince people to leave me alone. On the tapes, there was recommended reading material. I ordered them all from a local book store. I was reading again and listening to the tapes that had ridden shotgun with me for thousands of miles. The thirst for knowledge, answers, was coming back. But where was the passion? Still elusive, I could get wrapped up in a conversation; wheels would turn. Yes, that could be done but, within a day or so, the excitement or passion was just gone. I kept asking people involved in my therapy, "Where is it? How come it doesn't stay? What's wrong with me?"

Well, everyone had their word or explanation for my word "passion". They were all close, but I knew I was missing that burning I felt in the pit of my stomach when a desire comes into being, and it sat there fueling the momentum that had pushed me through to the end of the project. It was gone, I couldn't make it come back. I was in mourning for this driving force.

One day, on my desk was a catalogue from my old-time friends, "Nightingale-Conant". A new tape series, "Core Passion". There was my word! Someone else thought it applied to the human drive mechanism as well. I made photocopies and typed a letter to my doctor with copies to everyone else who had looked at me quizzically. See, "passion", my word. My wonderful Dr. Wardner was quick to respond, stating he couldn't write a prescription for it, but it might help me. Once again, the battle with self-confidence kicked in. I often said, "I must speak Martian now " because often people didn't understand me. Was I writing in Martian, also? How come my doctor didn't understand my letter? I didn't want a prescription for those tapes. I didn't need those tapes. I understood passion. Mine was lost, and I couldn't find it.

I was on the phone. I didn't want a phone conversation. I wanted an appointment. I'd pay the $40.00, but I also wanted to feel that he really understood. Appointment made, I called the others to see if they knew what I meant. Marilyn knew, but my Pastor misread it, also. Maybe it was a man thing. Maybe it was also not knowing me very well. How was I supposed to regain the self-confidence I once had in abundance when every time I tried, I ended up explaining to someone just what I meant? Would it ever get better? I knew the one thing I could <u>not</u> do was hold onto the negative of this situation. Maybe I had to let go. If others didn't understand, that would have to be okay. I well knew the feeling that was absent in me. I'd know if it came back. But I also resolved that if it didn't, I could still watch Danny grow into manhood. I could still hug those precious grandchildren, applaud the success of the other children, and slide my foot over and feel Doug on the other side of the bed at night, or hold his hand over coffee in the morning. Did the rest really matter? No, it didn't. I let it go, something I'd never been able to do easily before, but I just opened my arms and released it. Once the frustration left, it cleared the way for reason.

My neurosurgeon, Dr. Thomas, was on the phone. The MRI's I'd had since leaving the hospital were still inconclusive. Now, he wanted an angiogram. I'd have to stay overnight to be sure there was no bleeding, but he hoped that would give him the information he needed. While I was in the hospital, he was one of my least favorite people. I didn't like him--his bedside manner, nothing about him--but since going home, my perspective had changed and maybe that affected the way he talked to me. He even laughed during our conversations now. I also had cooperated through two MRI's, with the help of my new-found friend, valium. At least with the angiogram, they wouldn't be sending me down a tube the size of a drain tile. I could do that.

Doug checked me into the hospital, and they prepped me for the routine. On Sunday, the Pastor asked the congregation to "pray for Sue as she goes alone into the lab" for that procedure. From the pew, I had to respond, "but I won't be alone. I'm never alone". There was a new peace now that flooded my being. I'd never be alone again. I didn't remember ever being concerned before, but there is a new peace when faith finally settles in.

The technician was wonderful as he threaded the tube that would carry the dye up through the artery in my leg toward the brain. He must have been a teaching fellow because he was very patient with all my questions. He prepared me for all the feelings, and we were off and running. He even reran the tape and let me see the fireworks display as the dye shot through the right hemisphere of my brain, shooting toward the right frontal area that had been impacted by the blood. Well, no one could ever accuse me of not having a brain, or only half of one--I'd seen the film. Might not always work quite right these days, but there was one there.

Test over, it was back to my room to lie still for awhile. I did, for a while but not long. Because I'd been able to do this test without drugs, one of my favorite policyholders was in a room across the hall whom I wanted to visit, I got up! Besides, wanted a cup of coffee and a cigarette!

Being up and about and doing so well when the doctor made his rounds early evening, he decided I could just go home. He'd do the paperwork. He also remembered my trip to the Red Lobster. While he was in the process of writing the discharge order, Doug got a phone call from our daughter, Denise.

Danny had been in an accident. He had rolled his truck. Dad was to come right away. Although the conversation had included the fact that Danny was okay except for a bump on his head, Doug was still in a state. I was not going home. I was to stay in the hospital where they could watch me and he would take care of Danny. No arguments, that was the end of it. The doctor and I both said okay. Doug left. I needed to just touch and talk to Danny. We had both worried about this sort of thing from the day Danny had taken his truck out alone for the first time. Now, it had happened. Verbal assurances weren't enough for Doug. I drew once again on my faith.

Other than a little bump, Danny was okay. The truck was a total given its age, but the rollbar and seatbelts had kept both boys safe. Believing as always that sometimes good comes from bad, maybe this would show Danny just how fast it can happen, even to "good" drivers and make him more alert, more cautious. I think it has, but it also added to Doug's storehouse of bad things happening to us. When would the shoe drop again--Danny's accident, Doug's heart surgery, Grandma's falls and T.A.'s and the continuing decline of old age, my illness, now another accident. He felt we only got reprieves to once again gather strength for the next event. Now that I was able to read more than the short, inspiring vignettes from the encyclopedia of Robert Fulghum, All I Ever Needed to Know, I Learned in Kindergarten, I now read about dysthymia in the book, When the Blues Won't Go Away", by Robert Hirschfeld, M.D. Dysthymia: meaning lack of humor, sense of joy, the absence of the ability to cope with depression and pain.

Comes from two Latin root words, "painful soul/broken belief system". Developing humor skills can often help to move us along and through a hurting place. I believe sometimes just finding a way to get us outside and away from ourselves, putting a psychological distance between us and the pain can help move us along. It wasn't until just recently when I saw Doug, for the first time reach out to others, that I began to realize how very little I had tried to give Doug over the years. I read; I listened to tapes; I attended seminars and workshops; I got pro active; I went in search of the nourishment my mind, body and soul needed; but I failed to grab his hand and pull him along with me.

> After a while you learn the subtle difference between
> holding a hand and chaining a soul,
>
> And you learn that love doesn't mean leaning and
> company doesn't mean security,
>
> And you begin to learn that kisses aren't contracts and
> presents aren't promises,
>
> And you begin to accept your defeats with your head
> up and your eyes open, with the grace of an adult, not
> the grief of a child,
>
> And you learn to build all your roads on today because
> tomorrow's ground is too uncertain for plans.
>
> After a while you learn that even sunshine burns if you
> get too much.
>
> So plant your own garden and decorate your own soul,
> instead of waiting for someone to bring you flowers.
>
> And you learn that you really can endure . . . that you
> really are strong,
>
> And you really do have worth.
>
> --Anonymous

CHAPTER 21

My little Jewish friend, Marilyn, the one who makes miracles happen, decided that bowling was a normal thing people do. Those with head injuries were people, and they deserved to do normal things (differs greatly from "Loonie Logic"). So after weeks of meetings, she had put together an afternoon bowling league with patients from the surrounding facilities making up the teams.

Since Doug had bowled for years, knew all the rules, and was great at the technical stuff (Sue's logic), I volunteered him to be secretary for that league. He thanked me profusely the first two weeks in words I don't think I'd better write. But by the third week, it was all beginning to gel. Often with head injury, repetition is the key. They began to really know what was expected. They were ready to bowl when it was their turn, money was out and ready for collection, and many made the long walks over to tell Doug that they did well or they had gotten a strike. He cared enough to be there; they cared that he knew they did well.

Reciprocity--what goes around, comes around. I could see in his face, as he told me of how well it was going and of the differences in a few, that his spirit was getting nourishment. I'd looked out after my own for so long. I had not pushed him to become involved, but, now that he was, maybe we'd get a healing there, another small, but not a minor, miracle.

We had pushed Danny into normal situations through regular school classes and activities, through Choi Kwang Do in the community, his fundraising for Cystic Fibrosis, a part-time job, and through family trips. All our efforts for Danny had helped. We had now been given an opportunity to make a difference, not only in our lives, but the lives of others as well. Marilyn hadn't said a word this time; but once again, she'd been our guide.

A broken belief system, life often batters the one we have, but each of those occasions that bring us down also gives us the opportunity to get back up and I have always believed that life is often all about living up to those challenges. Our attitude, not our aptitude, determines our altitude. Doug had problems with that, and today still struggles with seeing the joys, counting the blessings. C. W. McCabe recommends making a "Joy List". We made an appointment with each other to sit down and do one recently. I'd recommend it. Even when things are the darkest, if you look hard enough, there often is a glimmer of light out there. And it doesn't have to be the light at the end of the tunnel according to Murphy's Law, the sign of an oncoming train. It can be the flicker of your own pilot light of faith and hope, and each passing day helps it burn stronger and brighter.

McCabe said that most of the people he proposed the "Joy List" to had trouble coming up with more than three things. Doug had six, and I had ten. Well, I really had nine that could be counted as things--the grandchildren, my children, friends, my faith--but I finished number nine, and I just could not resist putting down "talking", about all of the above. Made me smile, and that's what I think the "Joy List" is all about.

We often set ourselves up for feeling alone by drawing back and cutting off family and friends while we wallow in this awful mess we think we're in. Older people often start limiting their world, and, as they do, the decline comes faster. If we limit our worlds, our hope and spirit can do the same thing; and as it withers, so do we and those around us. I couldn't do that. The nucleus of my family extended to our church family, those involved with head injury, the family our business had become over the years, the insurance women all over the country, as well as people in our community that I cared very much about. They had held me up so often, as I had tried to do for them in the past and I let them hold me up again. Sometimes I think we're selfish when we deprive people who really want to help from helping. They need to feel good, too.

Cards and letters which had been read in the hospital, but not remembered, were once again read and cherished and, finally, were placed in scrapbooks, <u>this</u> time, for Mom. Some friendships are extra special. When I reread a letter from my friend, Dee, I cried, partly because while my mind had been in Indiana, I subjected her to a lot of verbal abuse. But she, like a true friend, kept coming back to visit me in the hospital, as she had from the beginning. I treasure her friendship as I do many.

Much like the man who seeing a hungry man, fed him. When the man asked his name so he could one day repay him, the benefactor said, "You need not repay me for this meal. If you see someone in need, you help them. That will be my payment." The philosophy of "pass it on"; how often we can do that and, not only give something to someone else, but enrich our own inner treasury.

Dee passed back to me through her friendship what I had not knowingly handed her before. Maybe we are all supposed to be like runners in a relay race, passing the baton to others through our lifetime. Dee's letter passed the baton. I will pass it on.

Dearest Sue:

> The phone has been ringing for weeks now. Everyone wants to know how you are doing and sending their best wishes and thoughts. I know you have probably received hundreds of cards with good wishes. If ever anyone in this world was well loved by her friends - you're it! Yet, I know that there is one friend you have not yet heard from - mc . . . no excuse, just not able to find the right word or way in which to say what I felt I needed to say. So I sat and thought about how I had felt when everything was happening to me last year. I remembered how I wanted to talk to someone, but didn't know who to really talk to. I remembered crying buckets when no one was around. I know I wanted desperately to hold onto my husband, because he knew me and protected me and loved me no matter what - but he was working through his own grief and sometimes it seemed like it was all he could do to just get through the day himself. I was confused and my brain tired. I found myself praying a lot, but they often had things in them like - Why did You let this happen to me and to my family? God, I don't deserve this! They were moments of anger, fear and frustration . . . until one day the postman brought me a very special card, from a very special person - her name was Sue Hoppe.

I know you've sent a lot of people a lot of cards over the years. You should probably own stock in Hallmark! But this one card had a very special message in it. It helped me through a very dark time in my life, and I kept it close by. I have carried it in my purse, briefcase and suitcase. It has laid on my nightstand and serves to remind me of things I should not have forgotten. I thought I would share with you, what you once shared with me that meant so very much, and helped me through a tough year.

> **. . . I have thought about you so much these past few days and was going to call, but I know how sometimes it's easier to make your world smaller and not have to talk so much. I'm so sorry . . . You are a special lady. You certainly did not deserve to lose a dream . . . it's one of those times when you do lose a dream, but have to start working on another. <u>Keep in mind that in the same way a mother holds and comforts a small child, and promises all the hurt will pass, and it will get better, that God holds Mothers while they cry</u>. Those tears no one else can understand, that come from the soles of your feet, the hurt is so bad. But, He will be there! Let Him keep His arms around you, dear friend, as mine will be in thought. I'm here if you need me, and you're in my prayers.**

I know I told you thank you for the card, but I also know that I never told you how very special it was to me. It took your words to remind me that I was not alone. The Holy Spirit worked through you to remind me that God was with me, and that close and caring friends were with me. Just as they are with you now. The past year of my life has been greatly blessed, even though it has been a difficult struggle. I have new dreams now becoming realities. Barbie's adoption is being finalized this month. I wanted you to be one of the first to know of our good news! The new insurance agency is opening its doors in a few weeks, and I owe a great deal to you for that dream coming true! You encouraged me, mentored me and, most importantly, reminded me of my own faith when it was on some pretty shaky ground.

Whenever I feel really alone or hurting, I still conjure up your words that you wrote in my card . . . "God holds mothers while they cry." I have felt His arm around me, holding me and keeping me on the right track. One of my very favorite pictures has always been of

Christ the Shepherd with His flock, and the first song I ever learned to sing in Kindergarten at Holy Ghost Lutheran School was I AM JESUS LITTLE LAMB. I pulled the words out and looked at them today. I thought I would share them with you. I also looked up the Bible passages that inspired their writing. I decided that every time you sent a card like the one you sent to me, you must have been like Simon Peter, following God's command to "Feed my sheep". We have kidded a great deal this past year about being sheep in NAIW. I believe that NAIW was just one of His many flocks, and I'm sure glad we ended up in the same pasture!!! You have carried so many of us during tough times, and shared so much of yourself. I pray that you will find some small comfort in this "epistle"! I know that I have felt the strength of many prayers joining mine for your quick recovery back into the fold.

Please know, dear friend, that I care very much about you. If you need anything, you call me! If you need to talk, or just sit quietly with someone there, or to read to you, or whatever, you call me . . . anytime. The number again is 587-2062. The new office will be opening soon, and although the phones are not yet connected, the number there will be 457-9009. I will be stopping in to see you frequently, after all, someone has to keep you posted on the issues!

I can't think up any clever words of my own, certainly nothing that could mean as much as the ones you shared with me. So, I will close for now and leave you with the words to what as a child was my favorite song - maybe it'll become one of yours.

Yours in Christ and friendship,

Dee

These friendships that can hold you up remind me of a Reader's Digest article I read years ago about, of all things, Sequoia trees. It seems that these beautiful trees have roots which barely grow below the surface of the ground, but they grow tall and aren't blown over by the wind. As they grow in groves, their roots intertwine under the surface so that strong winds, when they blow, are unnoticed. They hold each other up.

People can be like that, too. Doug and I have managed for years to do that. Family, friends, neighbors, support groups become havens (groves, if you will) and when adversity hits you like gale force winds, you remain standing. The other thing these support systems allow the feeling that "they know I'm here", much the same comfort as the voice at the other end of the phone gave me when I came home from the hospital. They will offer comfort beyond measure. As you make your way along the road back, join hands, bring others along; it will be good for everyone and remember, laugh while you're doing it. A little internal jogging never hurt anyone.

Who would have thought, the day we met,
That it would last so long?
This friendship that has come to pass
Has grown to be so strong.

I know when I am laughing
You'll find the humor, too;
So each of life's absurdities
I tend to share with you.

You've held me in my sorrow;
I've held you in your pain.
We've shared each new tomorrow
Through sunshine, clouds and rain.

You are the one I turn to
In good times and in bad.
I love to hear your laughter, and
I hate it when you're sad.

I never had a sister, but
As near as I can tell
I couldn't love a sister more--
Nor nearly half so well.

Though I may have a lot of friends
Who help to see me through.
God never gave a greater gift
Than when He sent me you.

--Kathleen Randolph Conat

CHAPTER 22

Danny has just completed another battery of tests for a new neuro-psych evaluation, mostly with a smile on his face. We've been through physical evaluations and a Video Gait Analysis, and he endures the pain of the exercises, all with the same "no pain, no gain" attitude that has spurred him on for all these years. "Sen Sei", Japanese for teacher. In my mind is what this young man continues to do for me. Everyday he makes me smile. Everyday, by example, he encourages me to meet the problem head on, accept the challenge and not to go down in the "agony of defeat" when your only competitor is what's inside you. He is working hard to live up to, not my expectations for him, but those he has for himself--to be the best he can be. How much so many could learn from this child of mine. I'm sure there are many parents out there who watch their children fight valiantly for recovery or just to live another day. It may be painful to lose them forever or to lose the person they were to the never-never land of head injury, but how much richer we are to have had their incredible spirits, as if sent by the "angels", as part of our life's journey. How much richer we are when they hold our hand and guide us back to another day.

I take one day at a time, much slower now than before. I make time to let people know I care. I try and spend more time with family. I can now say "no". I've also learned to say, "I can't do that", and sometimes I really can't. If I generate the process from within myself, it's not a problem. If Doug puts a pile of folders on my desk and issues instructions, I lose track. I've learned compensatory strategies for me that allows him to tell me and leave, and then I struggle through on my own. It may never be the way it once was. I may never be able to juggle four or five projects, but it really doesn't matter anymore.

Since I started the recovery process, I've been chided for making light of brain damage, which is serious business. Brain damage is serious. All of us with it take it seriously. We go to therapy; we put things in place to help us function. We've struggled with the tests, dealt the best we could on any given day with what we've lost, who we were as compared to who we are now. Many have had severe losses, but then many people were and are born with the same deficits and they never will have had the opportunity of only a few years without the handicaps. At least we had some time. Should we not be thankful for that and then work to get back what we can and be the best that we can be now?

I said before I was not going to become this injury, and I'm not. I laugh and tap my forehead. The doctor says, "That's not funny." It makes me feel good, and I only do it in front of the so-called "normal people". I was once one of those, and I was not a happy person. I wanted the awards, the recognition. I needed to be the leader, or a better word may be "boss". I was truly a much more needy person before the "B" word than I am now.

When the computer in my head decided to short circuit and stop me in my tracks, it probably was the best thing that ever happened to me. The person who emerged came forth much like a butterfly bursts forth, able to fly away free, unhampered by the furry body. I was released from 47 years of old, taped messages.

Still determined to find the lost passion, finally Dr. Wardner (in self-defense) referred me to an old friend, Dr. James Papsdorf (who had once worked with Danny) for testing. The day the appointment arrived and after the traditional "How are you's", I began our session.

"Well, I think you should start a chart and then keep it as a sample of your cure rate," I told him. "I'm here to find my passion. We'll talk, and I'll leave, satisfied and cured."

Given our long acquaintance, Dr. Papsdorf smiled and listened and then said, "How so?"

I now knew where the passion had gone and it was never coming back. I didn't want it back because the old passion, the fire that drove me, was fueled by old baggage and by the anger that it caused. By God "taking the garbage out", he took the old resentment, hurts, rejection and the pain from childhood. Also, all the pain I had been bottling up for ten years because of Danny's injury, was GONE. What I thought was "passion" was all these things, probably externally being denied but internally, being converted to a very dangerous fuel which drove me, and probably chauffeured me right into the hospital bed. Well, it was gone now. "Thank you, God." And I didn't want it back. For years, I must have been treating the symptoms, not the problem, by the bandaid effect of being too busy to think. Now that I was not going to be allowed to do that, and I couldn't if I wanted to, I would work through it.

With many head injuries, the areas of damage are scattered. In the insurance business, we have said for years that a liability lawsuit has a shotgun effect--so do many TBI's. I was fortunate to only lose a few thousand cells in the right frontal lobe. Now that I was finally in tune with myself, I could let it go. I did not want the old me back, but I did want to know as much as I could about the new me.

The new person still carried with her a natural curiosity and a thirst for knowledge, which showed up in the "Motivational Analysis Test". The new person still had a competitive drive, vigilance, an ego and the need for self-development. There was no longer a need for status or to be the dominant character in any performance.

I redid a test that I had taken (an identical one) several years ago and it did nothing to alter my theory. The Personal Profile System, developed by Performax Systems International, is used all over the country. As a coordinator for one of their other programs, I had these available to me to use for workshops. When I had taken the original test four years ago, I was unquestionably a high dominance personality. I wanted immediate results, challenges, authority, and was always questioning the status quo. I wanted action and often prompted it. Solving problems, a strong suit for that personality, may have been what drove me so hard with Danny. If it were, I'm grateful that all the garbage I'd collected for those 40 years prior to his accident was there, but now I like the currently described "influencing personality" that comes out "across the board" on the retest.

Motivating people, enthusiasm, entertaining, desire to help, participation in life, the sheer joy in being alive. How wonderful the change. How blessed I am to have been given all I needed once, and now all I need for the rest of my life. In the book, Man's Search for Meaning, by Frankel, he states that those who were confined and survived the Hell which was the concentration camps survived one of two ways--either by hate and anger or by appreciating life even in its cruelest form. How much we do of that sometimes escapes our recognition until we are forced by an incident in our life to review our life. I was enjoying life now more than I had in twenty-five years. I knew I was different and sought even more ways to prove it.

Into my life came Tom Killilea, a highly respected graphologist. I decided I should have my handwriting analyzed. Tom reinforced the enthusiasm, the willpower, curiosity, and persistence. The need to accomplish was still alive, as well as initiative and follow through.

He also brought to light characteristics which would not appear up on a standardized personality test. Difficulty making decisions--yes, that now was sometimes difficult. I never was one to sit on a fence or straddle the center of the road. I always felt the only thing in the middle of the road were the lines and dead animals; so you made a decision; and if it were wrong, you made another. Now I sometimes second guess myself, and I don't want to burn those bridges that before wouldn't have mattered because I would have said, "Oh, well, we'll build another." Now I'm not so sure I have the strength except when it comes to Danny.

When I get frustrated at my desk trying to figure out how to put something together, I get up and do something physical for ten or fifteen minutes. My office floor has been vacuumed so many times in the past few months; it's getting threadbare. The copy machine groans when I walk toward it. And we have plenty of clean coffee cups in the office now.

Because he said so many nice things about me, I paid the bill. When I look over the written results of the handwriting analysis and the personality testing, it helps allay the fear that I wouldn't be able to help Danny anymore or make my existence, this second chance at life, meaningful.

There are some days when I open my mail and read things like "Suzan Hoppe, Huge Success Potential, Released by Brain Wave Training, Study says Hoppe can learn to access same mental state as Edison, Freud, and Brahms"--that I'm glad I keep the office floor so clean because I'm on it laughing. There are other times when I truly hear what someone's saying because of the impact to the right frontal lobe (where the area of insight, intuition and hearing is for all of us) is now free of garbage, I am thankful. There was a song when I was a child that contained the words "live, love, laugh and be happy." I think I may have that made into a bumper sticker for my car and have someone else cross stitch it for my office (that is a skill I didn't have before, and I don't want now).

The doctor, however misguided I think he might be, was right when he said not everyone with brain damage can or wants to laugh about it. But those of us who have survived, who are able to, need to reach back to them. Those who are not so fortunate to have had an attitude adjustment can reach out also and encourage him/her to be the very best s/he can be. How do we know until we really go hunting for the person within, who might be there? I was and am pleased with the new me. Could the other new person maybe be a better person than the one who was taken away by the trauma? Throughout history, there were any number of people who, on the surface, gave many reasons to believe they would never do anything.

> Thomas Edison's teacher said it was useless for him to attend school.
>
> Abraham Lincoln was called a dreamer and told he asked foolish questions.
>
> Woodrow Wilson's parents were told not to put their sights too high because he was ten and couldn't read or write.
>
> Albert Einstein was called mentally slow.
>
> Carusso was told he had no voice.

> Louisa May Alcott was told that no one would ever purchase her stories.
>
> Sir Walter Scott was a cripple.
>
> Beethoven was deaf.
>
> Harriet Tubman, George Washington Carver, Martin Luther King, sound of mind and body, were born black.
>
> Burned and scarred, Glenn Cunningham set the record for running a mile.
>
> Franklin D. Roosevelt, crippled by infantile paralysis, became President of the United States. When asked once where he got the stamina to keep going and the will to keep trying to make changes, he responded by saying, 'You're looking at someone who worked for two years to be able to wiggle his big toe.'

Maybe, just maybe by the experience, by the effort, by the will to live and the joy in being alive, there are many more butterflies out there.

Some form of seizure activity is now plaguing Danny and interfering with his life. He is angry at the limitations that have now been put on him, but this eaglet, who has been trying desperately to leave the nest and soar with the grownups, does not feel powerless, does not feel that adversity has challenged him beyond his ability to endure. He's wanting answers and rightfully so. He deserves them, and we'll continue to press for them. Danny used to cheer as he was learning to walk, "You gotta want it, and you gotta want it bad". It is once again part of his vocabulary and once again I learn from him. How fortunate I am, how blessed I've been.

Written in Hebrew, sounds like:

Mahn ass stah

Ha Layla Ha Zay

Loosely translated, it means "Why should this day be any different from the rest"--a statement made in reply to my apology for keeping Danny's doctor so late one evening. From the Jewish faith, Christian Old Testament, it comes from the time of Passover. We know why it was different then. In business, when office hours are often 10 or 12 hours instead of 8, it takes on yet another meaning. When we apply it to those recovering from an insult to the brain, it takes on quite another.

For me, as I recover, every morning that I wake up is a special gift, a day to do with as I please, to give, to take, to help, to care, to grow and maybe inspire. Another day to laugh, hug grandbabies, encourage Danny, offer hope, and maybe be as much of the person I was as I want to be. All of us given the gift of life have the obligation to use each day to its fullest potential. It becomes an even greater obligation when, as a caregiver, patient advocate, parent or spouse of a person with a head injury (who, maybe, like me), couldn't remember five minutes, let alone what I was going to do with the day. A person whose emotions are out of control, and in that panic which blossoms into full bloom when confronted with that loss of control, can't begin to plan for a day either.

I needed, as many do, a strong, caring person to set the sails on my boat for that day, to chart its course. The charted course needs to enter new territories where learning and wellness can be found. On each venture out, as more goals are met, more successes discovered, the statement "Why should this day be different" can become a contradiction. It should be different because a goal was met. It may be only moving a finger slightly or blinking to turn on a computer screen, but it is different from the day before because this day can then become a celebration of that one inch of progress on the rehab mile, and it is truly different from all the rest.

Shalom

GOD SAID NO

I asked God to take away my pride,
and God said NO.
He said it's not for Him to take away
but for me to give up.

I asked God to make my handicapped child whole,
and God said NO.
He said, her spirit IS whole,
her body is only temporary.

I asked God to grant me patience,
and He said NO.
Patience is the by-product of tribulation.
It isn't granted, it is earned.

I asked God to give me happiness,
and God said NO.
He gives blessings,
happiness is up to me.

I asked God to spare me pain,
and He said NO.
Suffering draws you apart from worldly cares
and draws you closer to Me.

I asked God to make my spirit grow,
and God said NO.
He said I must grow it on my own.
He will help with regular pruning.

I asked God if He loved me,
and He said YES.
He gave His only Son to die for me.
And that's why I will be in heaven with Him one day.

So I asked God to help me love others as
much as He loves me.
And He said: "Ahh! So you finally got the point."

EPILOGUE

It is my hope that sharing with you my family's trials through two brain injuries gives you some insight into this twist of fate which has now impacted yours. While I was in the hospital, there was one constant: Hanging next to my bed was a reprint of "Footprints". It is on just about everything now so I am sure you are familiar with it. That print hung in my home and my office and through Danny's recovery, and it comforted me during mine.

When I was close to finishing this writing, one morning I happened to look at "Footprints" hanging in my kitchen and thought of how we all, in one way or another, hope to leave footprints as we pass through this world. Footprints, aided or otherwise, leaving our mark for eternity on the sand of time.

Many who came before us have left their footprints: Women like Marilyn Spivak who, because of her daughter, started the National Head Injury Foundation. She took a step of faith and formed a strong coalition of families that provide information, caring, and a feeling of "I belong here." The support groups help cushion the pain and offer their hand to help us along the path we must now follow. Because many made it easier for those to come, it now becomes our charge to keep the path clear for those in the future. An unused path can soon become overgrown with weeds, and, if we've come through the fire, the walk from then on is even more important.

REFERENCE LIST

Books, tapes, and seminars can be food for the mind and the soul. If you haven't read these, you might want to give them a try.

When Bad Things Happen to Good People
When All You Ever Wanted Isn't Enough
By Rabbi Harold S. Kushner

Forgive and Forget
Caring and Commitment
By Lewis B. Smedes

The Be Happy Attitudes
Tough Times Don't Last But Tough People Do
By Robert Schuler

When It Hurts Too Much To Wait
By Larry Richards

Confidence
Bringing Out the Best in People
The Friendship Factor
By Alan Loy McGinnis

How To Be A No Limit Person
By Dr. Wayne Dyer

Making Miracles
By Dr. Pearsoll

You Can't Afford the Luxury of a Negative Thought
By John Rogers and Peter McWilliams

Quantum Healing
By Deepak Chopra, M.D.

When the Blues Won't Go Away
By Robert Hirschfeld, M.D.

Meditations for Women Who Do Too Much
By Anne Wilson Schaef

Your Attitude/Key To Success
By John C. Maxwell

All I Really Need To Know I Learned in Kindergarten
It Was On Fire When I Laid Down
Uh, Oh
And anything else this man ever writes. He has a wonderful gift of giving the reader perspective.
By Robert Fulghum

Encouragement - The Key to Caring
By Lawrence J. Crabb, Jr. and Dan B. Allender

Happiness is a Choice
By Barry Neil Kaufman

Many of our best speakers and motivators draw from the one book that we all have access to, that's been around through the ages. It offers wisdom, hope and inner peace. You might find solace in reading:

Psalm 40: 1 - 3
Psalm 34: 17, 19
John 14: 1 - 3
Deuteronomy 31: 6
Isaiah 41: 10
Psalm 32: 7
Hebrews 10: 36
Isaiah 26: 3, 4
Psalm 37: 7
Isaiah 41: 13
Psalm 4: 8
Isaiah 54: 10
John 14: 18
2 Corinthians 4: 17; 12: 7 - 10
Isaiah 40: 31
1 Peter 5: 7
Philippians 2: 3, 4
Psalm 16: 7, 8
Psalm 25: 9, 10
Matthew 7: 7, 8
Hebrews 11: 1
Romans 15: 13
Psalm 31: 24
James 1: 3

Proverbs 17: 17
John 15: 15
Psalm 119: 71
Matthew 5: 4
Romans 12: 15
Romans 8: 28
Proverbs 18: 24
Romans 12: 12
Galatians 6: 9 - 10
1 John 5: 14 - 15
Matthew 5: 14 - 16
Job 11: 18 - 20
Psalm 30: 5
Mark 11: 24
Matthew 11: 28 - 30
Proverbs 17: 22
1 Corinthians 13: 7
Matthew 18: 20
Mark 4: 24
1 Corinthians 9: 24, 25
Proverbs 18: 24
John 15: 13
1 Corinthians 7: 7; 13: 7

Thoughts for a Month of Mondays ...

I don't know when Mondays started getting a bad rap but I do know they are often defined as not only blue, but unpleasant. When you must go through an injury or an illness – maybe your own, maybe that of a family member, you greet many of those days as if they were a Monday. Hope these thoughts for a Monday will help you to keep looking forward to a coming Tuesday, even if your month of Mondays may be more than thirty days.

Monday 1

A New York businessman on a trip to the bayou country of Louisiana stood and watched a young boy catching crawdads (crayfish) and tossing them into a bucket. As the bucket filled he became concerned that some of the catch would crawl back out so he walked over and asked the young man why he didn't have a cover on the bucket. The lad looked up and just smiled. Probably figured this Northerner didn't know much to begin with. "Don't worry Mister, these ole' crawdad's won't go nowhere, ain't no need for a cover". With this said he continued to place his catch in the bucket.

Our businessman continued to be puzzled by the lack of a cover and strode over to peer into the bucket. As he watched the growing pile of Crawdads he also saw why there was indeed NO COVER NEEDED.

The larger stronger crawdads were in fact climbing over the smaller ones and vainly attempting to go up and over the side of the bucket. But the ones that were now content with their lot in life which was now to be someone's dinner, would reach up and pull the bigger ones back down into the bucket with them, and their acceptance of their fate.

People can, as they live their lives after a traumatic injury or illness, be like the crawdads. They can resign themselves to stay at the bottom of life's bucket or they can make the attempt to go over the wall, being mindful of those who will attempt to keep them in a state of complacent resignation.

Being someone's dinner never appealed to me, and I hope as you replay this scenario you will develop the strength to push away from you, those people who will attempt to pull you back into the bucket of despair and hopelessness. Gumbo may make a good dinner, but the stew that can come from a psychological pot which contains none of the flavorings of life, offers no food for the mind, the body, or the soul.

Monday

2

When defining humor with head injury you might want to do it this way.

H: Heart - The capacity to love, to have courage and compassion.

U: Unity - Unity within the family structure to take the problem seriously, themselves lightly.

M: Method - For a systematic effort to overcome the pain, the despair. Be open but don't deny it.

O: Order - Bring order into your world by taking control of how you choose to see it.

R: Relax - Days come and go in spite of you. Meet each new one as a friend. See it as the doorway to a new opportunity. Maybe a miracle.

Monday 3

How we change or fix our attitudes makes the difference in not only ourselves, but our special family member, as well as the rest of our family. When our vision of the future becomes like that of a gold miner, we don't see all the dirt that has to be moved to find the gold, we keep our vision focused on finding the gold. The focus must always be, finding the gold.

We have just experienced another Olympic Games, and we saw many people strive for the gold medal. Some received Silver, some Bronze, and many received no medal at all. But, they did go home knowing that they were good enough to get there, and had the opportunity to compete.

Without the vision they held before themselves the many months before the actual competition, all the months of training and without the belief that they had a chance, many would not have continued.

As a caregiver or as a survivor we have our own special Olympics on a daily basis. Our goals are to have the best recovery programs available. To always hold in front of us the vision of what can be. To run the race, to break a record, to bring a new meaning to a life, to see physical and mental growth. Have the vision, go for the GOLD.

Monday 4

In C.S. Lewis' "The Chronicles of Narnia", as the warring between good and evil waged and approaching what would be the final battle, the Dwarfs after one particular encounter, announced that they were tired of hearing about Aslan, they wanted no more of Kings and other worlds. "The Dwarfs are for the Dwarfs". They marched away singing a queer little song to fend for themselves. They continued to do battle but they only fought against whomever they perceived threatened them most. The Dwarfs remained for the Dwarfs.

The Dwarfs were excellent archers and during the final battle they were able to fell many horses and riders before they were captured and then sent through the stable door.

Others who had passed through the stable door into the new land found colors more vibrant than any they had ever seen. The air was so clean, flowers smelled sweeter,fruit more delicious, everything was a wonderment. But the Dwarfs sat huddled in a tight little circle and when they were told to look around them at all the beauty, they could only respond, "What are you talking about" "It's dark, it smells bad, and all we have is each other. The Dwarfs are for the Dwarfs. Leave us alone!" Given the chance to experience good in their lives the Dwarfs chose to remain turned inward unto themselves. Afraid to let go of the world they had created, even though it was unpleasant, it was theirs, and it was certain.

We do that sometimes when our world as we created it, is changed by a head injury. We close ourselves off because we feel that no one knows the pain. We limit our world instead of trying to find ways to broaden it and bring in others. Open your heart and your mind, expose the pain, share the worry, let others help and guide you. There is no one unhappier than the person who has let their spirit become a Dwarf.

Monday 5

The marvelous richness of human experience would lose something of rewarding joy if there were no limitations to overcome. The hilltop hour would not be half so wonderful if there were no dark valleys to traverse.

"I have never believed that my limitations were in any sense punishments or accidents. If I had held such a view, I could never have exerted the strength to overcome them."

Helen Keller

If I use my favorite word " perspective", and look at my son's problem with his left side, the memory deficits, and then look at my own deficits and compare them to those Helen Keller overcame as well as the contribution to the world she made anyway, it's hard to get depressed. When I think of what the future can hold for Danny and me if we use what we have left to its fullest potential, it is truly exciting.

Monday 6

Why do I need a support group? George Eliot once wrote on friendship- "oh, the comfort, the inexpressible comfort of feeling safe with a person; having neither to weigh thoughts nor measure words but to pour them all out, just as is, chaff and grain together, knowing that a faithful hand will take and sift them, keeping what is worth keeping, and then, with a breath of kindness blow the rest away."

Alan Loy McGinnis from his book The Friendship Factor - "With these friends you make a real effort, and then you break the barrier and you go beyond. This is a fantastic thing - you go home and lie awake because so many facts in your mind and soul have been opened. It's a feeling of discovery that something here inside you seems to be growing opening and expanding."

Building friendships and relationships is something that has to be cultivated and worked on. Time, trust and transparency help to build these in support groups. Families caring for families. How nice it is to say, "I need time away, I'm so tired, so angry. This has been a terrible week." You can say anything and someone will respond, "I've been there, I understand, is there anything I can do?"

No two injuries are the same, but heartache, disappointment, anger, worry, the pain of the loss feels the same to everyone. A professional unless s/he has been there, really can't know no matter how hard s/he may try. The best education is by doing, having been there. How good it can feel to know you are not alone. Just to know someone does understand. To feel that something may not seem right but it is still okay.

If you don't belong to a support group, give serious thought to finding one. It may provide you with the nourishment you now need.

Monday 7

One of the Ten Commandments says, "Thou shalt not covet". Covet, to desire, to long for something that belongs to someone else. Right up there with "Envy" and "Desire". There are a number of words the Thesaurus will liken to the word "covet". But, the one word it doesn't use that I think it should, is "Enslave".

When we covet, or desire, or envy someone or something so strongly that we push aside everything else, how can we say we are free. We are now in bondage, held captive by a thought process that not only stunts our personal growth, but our emotional and spiritual growth as well. We become like the "Dwarfs" and limit ourselves.

Devise a few Commandments of your own. Thou shalt be the best you can be. Thou shalt have choices. Love yourself just the way you are, for God loves you.

Monday

8

Before my illness and now once again I am an avid reader of not only books but trade magazines, journals, medical information, and now even though it is not pleasurable for me, computereze. There was an article in a church newsletter by Dr. Norman R. DePuy of Newton Center MA, that I read and then re-read, cut out and have gone back to again and again from my pile of clippings wondering why? What is the catch phrase? In his piece he wrote about seeing a hitch-hiker with a placard saying Newton or Miami Beach. He then pondered that seldom in life do we have such a broad choice of options.

That was the hook in the article. Many times our lives seem dead-ended. We're in a job or a marriage or a family situation which seems to close down our life, keeps us from hope, and makes us depressed with the lack of choice. The one thing that we do have going for us can only be likened to the pilot light of a stove. It is always there like that tiny flame that ignites the burner, the tiny flame, the flicker of hope. As long as our bodies can draw a breath, the sometimes almost imperceptible flicker at any time can burst into a flame. The door to new possibilities is not closed forever, and just when we are in the extremes of despair, we may find that surprisingly, the opposite has become the case.

With all the failings of man and his actions, the miracle of the human body and its reserves is unquestionable. If we can manage to fan that flicker of hope into a larger, and larger flame, then all through our lives and the lives of those we love will have as broad a choice, unlimited options, as the hitch-hiker and his placard.

Monday 9

Three men were breaking rocks, and a contractor was going to hire one of them. He went up to the first one and asked. "What are you doing"? "I'm breaking rocks" was the reply. He went to the second man and asked him the same question. "I'm breaking rocks that will be used in a building". When he asked the third man he anticipated the same answer. The third man said "I'm building a cathedral." Which one would you hire? Which one are you?

As a caregiver you are every inch a stone mason as any of these men. The persons recovering from a traumatic brain injury must start rebuilding their lives with a firm foundation. They can be what you help them to be. Don't they deserve the opportunity to be a cathedral?

Monday 10

Somewhere on a dairy farm, two frogs happened to fall into a bucket of milk which had not yet been processed. The one frog was in a state of panic. "We'll never get out of here you know," he said. To which the other replied "just keep paddling". "It's too far to the top to jump", "just keep paddling". "The milk isn't thick enough to sit on," "just keep paddling". "We're never going to get out of here." "Just keep paddling" was once again the reply. Our first little frog kept up the lamenting until finally he just gave up and sank below the top, never to be heard again. The other persistent little frog just kept on paddling and by morning found himself sitting on top of a rather large pat of butter.

After months of therapy, not only the head injured but often the families, give up and quit. The turning of the milk to butter not only seems a long way off but sometimes it seems like an impossibility. We hear about STRESS, BURNOUT, MENTAL FATIGUE, EXHAUSTION. there are many names given to those things we feel after we've pushed so hard for so long. There is nothing wrong with feeling any of these, but we have to find a way to get past them, and to keep paddling with a new attitude and a new perspective.

Our surviving frog did just what he needed to do. He controlled the situation instead of letting the situation control him. Why not give it a try.

Monday
11

The devotion of a parent to a child- the combination of protecting them and pushing them out of the nest - is the epitome of leadership, and it is the best example of motivating without manipulating."

Alan Loy McGinnis

Sometimes forgetting a child has a handicap is the best thing we can do for him/her. A mother bird knows she must push the baby from the nest or it will never fly. Our injured children can never learn to function in the world if we don't push them out into it. We must realize that they may come back to us bruised and beaten up, and that we must then provide them with a temporary safe haven, but only temporary. Loving them demands, that we force them to recognize and learn to use their wings.

Monday
12

I was raised on a farm, and then as well as the now of many years later, I've watched herds of cows either standing or lying, all facing the same direction. Although I've noticed this I always figured it was just a "Cow thing" and didn't waste any more time dwelling on it.

A while ago I heard a speaker on the survival of cattle during the blizzards which often happen out on the western plains speak regarding which breed is most apt to survive. The ranchers that raise cattle lose large numbers unless they are able to get men out to round them up and drive them to shelter because the cattle will turn their backs to the storm and walk away from it.
In doing so they often find themselves in box canyons, up against a fence, or other object that blocks their forward motion. Once in this predicament they stand there, the storm overcomes them and many freeze to death.

Herefords on the other hand will not walk with their back to the storm. Instead, they turn and walk towards the snow, and into it. They keep a forward movement until the storm subsides or they walk out of it. Whatever, the cattle owners have in fact lost less of their herd.

Maybe there is a message there for people, especially those of us who now face a trauma. When adversity is blowing in our faces, maybe the wisest thing for us to do is not turn our backs and try to get away from it, only to have it overtake us. Instead meet it head on. Having identified the threat, we could be putting ourselves in a much better position to overcome IT. Keep a forward motion. Keep looking for the new. Advocate for the special person in your family, fight for the rights due them, and who knows how far you will have come when the storm subsides.

Monday 13

A friend of mine widowed a year ago just ended a relationship with a man who was found to be, in a very short period of time, not a knight in shining armor.

This friend is also trying to determine what she will collect. Many people have their pet things, cats, clowns, bears etc.

I have just written her and suggested that she should start collecting frogs. Remember the princess who had to kiss the frog to find her prince? As in real life, not fairytales we often have to kiss a lot of frogs to find the prince. Once found though, we may feel it was worth the effort.

In working through rehabilitation the tasks may feel like kissing so many frogs. Meet them on your terms; do the work, give them a kiss, and let being the very best you can be, be your prince.

Monday 14

Alan Loy McGinnis in his book "Confidence" tells about Yoshihko Yamamoto of Nagoya City, Japan. When he was six months old his parents learned that he suffered from hydrocephalus, an abnormal amount of fluid on the brain. Physicians told his parents that their child would probably be mentally retarded. A hearing loss complicated his speech and his IQ was tested at about 47. Things did not look too good.

Then Yoshihiko acquired a new teacher, Talashi Kawasaki who liked his new pupil and he worked at building a trusting relationship. Soon Yoshihiko learned to copy his letters and write his name. He also began to copy pictures from books.

One day Yoshihiko drew a sketch of the Nagoya Castle. The sketch reminded the teacher of a print so he had his young charge transfer the picture to a wood block and encouraged him in the art of printmaking. Soon he was winning art contests and selling his work. He still requires help with daily living skills and must maintain an ordered life, but he goes to school, works on his prints, and sees that which he can accomplish bring joy and beauty to many people.

Is it important that Yoshihiko does not have a high IQ? Is it important that he has limitations? No, the important thing is that he is doing the best he can with what he has, A thing that some with very high IQ's fail to do on a daily basis.

As we watch special persons in our lives struggle to get a foothold, maybe part of our job is to take the responsibility to see that they capitalize and maximize the abilities they have. Assist them in parlaying those skills to their highest potential. When we do this we give to them something that we cannot place a value on. We give them a sense of self worth, as well as meaning and quality to their life.

Monday 15

The Chinese language does not have a word for problem. Their word translates into decision point. The point between crisis and opportunity.

I would suggest to you that maybe while you're dealing with a traumatic brain injury, you remove the word "problem" from your vocabulary and adopt for yourself the term "decision point".

Once the crisis of life and death has passed, everything from that point on is an opportunity.

Monday 16

A word I've heard used recently by several speakers is "serendipity". I did a little research and found out that Horace Walpole coined that word in 1745. It came from a fairy tale about the Princes of Serendip, which is now Ceylon. The princes went in search of treasures but rarely found what they were searching for. Instead they would often find far greater treasures. Maybe they were being guided by a greater power who knew what was best for them.

The past gives us many references to errors and failures which worked out better for the person or the world. Think about Columbus, Madame Currie, Jonas Salk. Look at all we've benefited by space research, and how medicine, when looking for one thing, often finds the answer for another.

Serendipity, to learn to dip into life with serenity. To learn to trust that our journey on the road to recovery, not one we would have chosen to travel, may be leading us. Maybe new insight, maybe to be part of a miracle.

There may be days when you'll hate where you are; I did. But we must always keep in mind that maybe, just maybe, there is that higher power which has something much better in store for us than that which we had gone in search for. Keep dipping into life with serenity.

Monday 17

Rabbi Harold S. Kushner writes, "Job needed sympathy more than he needed advice, even good and correct advice....He needed friends who would permit him to be angry, to cry and to scream, much more than he needed friends who would urge him to be an example of patience and piety to others. He needed people to say, (yes what happened to you is terrible and makes no sense,) not people who would say, "cheer up Job, it's not all that bad."

When you're living the pain of coma, of head injury, it IS that bad. I hid in the bathroom from the well-meaning social worker who wanted to pat my hand and see tears, who wouldn't allow me to rage against the pain.

If you have a friend who needs to let the anger out and move past it, please allow him/her to do so.

Monday

18

Andrew Costello states: "Some people speak up and let difficult people know exactly how they feel." They fight back. Because "fight" has hostile overtones, perhaps it is not the best word to use here. "Assertiveness" might better describe what is meant. In any case fight is the opposite of flight. Instead of holding back and keeping silent in the presence of a difficult person, we speak up and let him or her know exactly where we stand.

Please speak up to family, friends, to the medical community. The one thing the brain-injured person needs as much as air, food and water is an advocate who can see that the injured is provided with those things they would have chosen, were they able.

Monday

19

One thing, or maybe it's two things a family new to head injury must do, is determine what you have control over and what you don't. Set the don'ts aside, then determine how you will win the race to wellness with "just to finish" your goal.

Making up your mind means you're halfway there.

I like to pick on golfers. My husband is a golfer so I'm allowed. Now many of them understand this principle early on, much like the foursome that played at the local club every Thursday.

Their lead golfer returned home much later one Thursday afternoon than was usual. He was red faced and obviously exhausted. His by then distraught wife questioned his being late. "Why were you so long? Why didn't you call? "Well you see Dear, Bob had a heart attack on the third hole. From then on it was hit the ball and drag Bob, hit the ball and drag Bob."

Well I guess that's better than the golfers in Florida who recently just left a man lay there; but the point is, they were determined to finish the game.

You have already all you need (right inside you) to finish this race to wellness. Hang in there; make up your mind to finish.

Monday 20

Since we talked about Golfers last Monday, let's continue. You probably have heard the story of the Heavenly Golf Game.

Jesus and Moses and this old guy in

ragged knickers were playing golf.

Moses addressed the ball. His drive curved and headed for the water. He held up his hands the water parted before the ball and it rolled up and onto the green, three feet from the pin.

Jesus addressed the ball, his drive also curved toward the water. He held up his hands, the ball sprouted feet, walked on top of the water, up on the green and stopped, two feet from the pin.

Now the old guy ambled over to the tee. Hit the ball. As it landed a gopher grabbed the ball and started to run. An eagle swooped down, caught the gopher in its talons and soared into the air. A bolt of lightning struck the eagle in the tail feathers. It dropped the gopher; the gopher hit the ground, the ball popped out of its mouth and into the cup. Hole in one!

Jesus looked over at the old man, then slapped him on the shoulders and said "great shot Dad!"

Now we may as families never have that kind of divine intervention, but remember, you don't see a miracle unless there is a problem first.

Monday 21

Sometimes our perspective of life becomes skewed when we use our personal frame of reference to judge the world.

When our love of laughter and the ability to love, to care, is not what the world gives us back, our world becomes a painful residence.

We must be vary careful during this time when we feel no sense of joy in being alive, that we continue to strive to separate ourselves from the event and find even a little joy in small things.

Studies have shown that 73% of all adult cancers onset is after a significant loss experience which we may perceive as unmanageable. Look for a way to manage it. Your injured family member, the rest of your family, and the world, needs you well.

All of life truly is a series of choices. Make yours to love, to laugh, to live.

Monday 22

Disability, the absence of ability. Handicapped, is that a cap with a hand on it? Is it one you grab because its handy?

I have problems with both of these terms. Disabled, in respect to what. Handicapped, applying how? Handicapable, too catchy. Nitpicking? Yes. I know it's a term designed lump all people with one limitation or another into one category, but what really bothers me is that either one seems to accentuate the negative rather than the positive. It also judges many of us against a norm. Who decided that norm? Were they right?

Do what you can, the best you can, and let those "the norms" live with some of their own self-imposed limitations.

Monday 23

Life is not now, nor has it been for many of us, a bowl of cherries. On any given day it can be more like the "pits".
Some days can be a real test to some and a more than real test to others. But it is life and that in my opinion is a whole lot better than the alternative.

As a survivor I would suggest to you that you don't allow anyone to make "YOU" the injury. It was serious; it is serious, and it must be taken seriously. Address that issue, meet it as a friend, and move beyond it.

I was not the brain damage. It was to become a very real part of my life, and I deal with it daily one way or another. But, it is only a small part of me, and I refuse to let it dampen my joy in being alive.

It's not easy to gain that perspective. I had a few problems with it. Moreso, because I had let a number of things grow in importance out of proportion to their real importance in my life, or the whole scheme of things.

Keep looking at the cherries! And when you do you will continue to be a very real value to family, to friends, and most importantly to yourself, and the world.

Monday 24

Critical care is a thing of the past. Hospital post acute care over. The patient and the family begin the reintegration to home and the community. Well-meaning people and those not so well meaning can say hurtful things about the person who may walk, talk, or think slowly.

More than once with Danny I recalled a story about Winston Churchill and his lifelong adversary Lady Astor. One time she confronted Sir Winston with the fact that he was not only drunk but disgusting. Never at a loss for words Sir Winston responded, "I may be drunk but you're ugly, and I'll be sober in the morning."

Made me smile then, makes me smile as I write it now. You can't change those people, but you can change how you react to them, which will ultimately make your recovery process easier. Find your own Sir Winston story and hold it close.

Monday 25

A couple of years ago, Louisiana had more than its share of rain and many areas became flooded. When the rains first started, they were being observed by an old man who sat on his porch and watched the rain come down and the flood waters rise until they were at his top step. When a row boat came by and offered to transport him to dry land he refused to go, saying "no thank you, the Lord will take care of me". Soon the water covered the front porch and our old man was forced to sit on the window sill. A motorboat came by and offered him a ride to higher ground, but once again the offer of assistance was refused and the boat driver heard again, "God will take care of me".

Well I'm sure you know by now that the water kept rising and the old man kept going higher and higher until he was sitting atop the roof. A helicopter hovered over head and they offered a basket on a rope to him, to carry him to safety. "no thank you, the Lord will take care of me" was once again his parting words to the would-be rescuers.

The water kept rising and the old man had no-where to go. After drowning he found himself in front of St. Peter and demanded an audience with God. When granted he demanded to know why, after all the years of being faithful, of believing, of always trying to be a good person, God had let him drown without trying to save him. When he finally had raged long enough he fell silent. In the silence God responded: "I did try to save you. I sent a row-boat, a motor-boat, and a helicopter."

Often we are presented with opportunities of which we can't see the value because we get in our own way. Making changes, taking a different direction, having to make a critical decision, all involve risk. Just maybe when we look at the risk we should put the alternatives IF we DON'T on the other side of the scale for proper balance.

Monday 26

M. Scott Peck in his book *People of the Lie*" states: "Having considered the relationship between evil and stress it is appropriate to comment on the relationship between goodness and stress. He who behaves nobly in the easy times - a fair weather friend so to speak - may not be so noble when the chips are down.

Stress is the test of goodness. The truly good are they who in the tie of stress do not desert their integrity, their maturity, their sensitivity."

The stress that head injury puts on parents, marriages, families, and siblings, cannot be denied in light of the overwhelming statistics. But if we are forewarned we can also be forearmed and not get blindsided by stress at a time when we need all the love, caring and support we can get.

No pain, not even the pain of death, equals the pain of the unresponsive loved one. But where statistics bear out the effects of stress, they also bear out the fact that most of those loved ones will return to us. Hang in there.

Monday 27

Discipline as defined by Webster is: "Training which corrects, molds, strengthens, or perfects. Rule or system of rules affecting conduct or actions."

Discipline is crucial to finding a way to sustain the human spirit, to move beyond the emotional numbness that can take over your psyche, when you find you're less of a person, less than you were before. It had been good once and if you can GET THROUGH THIS ONE DAY and then get through the one day which is tomorrow as well as the tomorrows ahead, one day at a time, each day will bring you one step closer to being that person of value in your own eyes. Maybe even of more value because of the experience.

Monday 28

One of the insights into myself I was allowed following my anuerysm was, as I took a new look at what I had thought to be important before, it now became insignificant to what I thought was important now. Doors close to us, but new doors open, often providing pathways to new challenges and answers to problems.

I had the opportunity to really see prayers answered. I got to be the participant in a miracle, as well as witness to two others. I also believe that even with the things I can't do: deal with numbers, consolidate outside information, process things as quickly as before, have limited energy, my loss of confidence in myself, I am far better off than those who can't or won't recognize that they also may have some.

People who lack understanding, compassion, the ability to respond to the needs of another human being; people who use and abuse others, and those who never bother to look deeper into a person than the body that presents to the world, are the people who really need help.

Enjoy and love your special person and feel compassion and forgiveness to those who have a handicapped soul.

Monday 29

The medical community has defined and named the emotional response to the survivors of the concentration camps of wars the KZ Syndrome and PTSD.

I can't tell you what KZ stands for but the PTSD means Post Traumatic Stress Disorder. I believe this occurs in families who have found themselves on the Brain Injury Battleground. When it hurts so bad that the only way we can get through the day is to kick in the numbing response, we're going to be in trouble if we don't find someone to help us learn coping mechanisms.

I also know that building a strong support system for yourself, or helping to build one for someone else helps. Being allowed to voice the pain, share the hurt helps. Using humor can also be a psychological medication that takes the edge off the pain. Don't wait until it's too late to start addressing the issue of stress.

Monday

30

John Powell states: "The first thing that love must do is communicate these three things: I truly care about you. I really want your happiness and I will do all I can to assure it. You are a uniquely valuable person".

How important it is that from the first moment of injury we do just that for the now-special person in our lives. It becomes even more important when that uniqueness has changed and s/he feels s/he has become a stranger in a strange land.

As a family member we need to go one step further and also become their anchor in reality. We must also become a buoy for their spirits even when our own are failing. Keep in mind that time is often the rescuer to everyone.

Monday

31

When I was a teenager one of the things I liked to do, and it only cost a nickel then, was to play the pinball machines.

Whether it is recovering from, or aiding the recovery from a Traumatic Brain Injury, your life can often become like that of the ball bearing in the pin ball machine.

The flipper sends the ball to the top and as it comes back down bells ring, it falls in holes to be popped back out, shoots off at an angle to be bounced off a bumper and heads in a new direction. The ball bearing seeking its own direction is often cut off by obstacles, and when it really thinks its home free, someone hits the flippers and goes right back to the top to start the process all over again.

There will be days when your world may resemble that of the pinball maze. But, there will also be days when the lights flash, bells ring, and you will rack up a winning score.

Monday

32

There is no correct way to grieve, but there is a healthy grief process.

1. Denial - It buys time to prepare for the inevitable, and sometimes causes withdrawal and isolation.

2. Anger - A person may take this out on friends, family, medical staff.

3. Bargaining - Sometimes trying to make a deal with God.

4. Depression - Numbness. Now you start dealing with the loss.

5. Acceptance - Not necessarily happy, but a sense of calm and peace.

When a person actually dies we move through this process and go on. With a head injury the grieving process is more complicated.

1. The family member is still alive, but different. That complicates the process.

2. Bargaining - You do it over and over. A perpetual crisis causes tremendous stress.

3. When it is a child it is much harder because parents feel they have somehow failed.

4. In a non-death loss these stages are repeated over and over. Sometimes this is more difficult than a complete loss.

5. When someone dies everyone takes over and lets you grieve. When there is no death, well-meaning people say things like, "why are you so sad? At least s/he is still alive." They

don't realize a little part of you is dying daily.

With time and love you CAN complete this process. You will one day say good-bye to the person they once were, or could have been. You will then have room enough in your heart to welcome the new and equally wonderful person they have become.

Monday 33

My Grandfather was a farmer all his life, and when I decided many years ago to put in my first garden, Grandpa and I had many conversations. He told me to plant by the moon. He told me when to weed. He told me how to plant the rows. He also advised that although I should care for the seeds, and then the small plants, I should not baby them. He believed that if you babied the plants early on and did not allow them to establish a good root system, when the elements turned harsh during the growing season, the garden would be in trouble.

I would imagine that families are very similar to the plants in my garden. Those who weather the storm of Head Injury best, are those who had a pretty good root system going into it.

Monday 34

If there is any profession that likes abbreviations more than the medical profession I would have to guess it's that of insurance.

I dedicated months, years, to achieving through study and exams, the initials after my name. I even contemplated acquiring more. A favorite statement of mine used to be that I would study until I had as many initials after my name as were in it.

I have decided that given my hospital stay, the months in therapy, as well as the continuing recovery process I will confer upon myself three more sets.

Now in addition to:

AAI - Accredited Advisor in Insurance

AAM - Associate in Automation Management

CPIW - Certified Professional Insurance Woman

I have conferred on myself:

HBD - Had Brain Damage

CRS - Can't Remember Stuff

BELA - But Enjoys Life Anyway

Monday 35

My wonderful husband, the golfer, has a habit that is not so wonderful. I call it "catastrophizing". Whether its something he can't find, something he thinks he SHOULD have, COULD have, or WOULD have done, it soon becomes the most awful thing that could have happened to him. Car problems, office problems are often blown out of proportion. When we had all the children at home he was much more interesting than he is now. Now we do the same thing occasionally with the WHAT IF'S.

Some things are bad. Sitting in the hospital waiting room wondering if our tiny son would live was bad. I'm sure as I hovered near death, it was bad for him also. But, wailing and beating our breasts would not have made any of it better. Berating yourself doesn't change the past. Hindsight is the only kind that is 20/20. None of us can predict the future. In the hospitals you will learn what makes you cry. Make a conscious effort to find those things that will comfort you. Seek out the things that give you hope. Look for reasons to laugh. You'll be better for it.

Monday 36

Have you ever noticed that nothing is ever given any real credence until the scientific community has said "YES", it could have happened?

Noah's Ark is now a possibility. They have just reported that yes, the Red Sea could have parted.

After a recent study the research data ia in: 75% of all Americans pray at least once a week. Experiments have also shown that it is a real benefit to your health.

Seek a quiet place, ask for strength, but remember that you also need to be quiet--still and quiet long enough so you can hear the answer.

Monday 37

One of the qualities found to be consistent in all those who successfully survived the POW camps, was their ability to retain their sense of self and maintain the feeling that they had some control over their lives. Despite the fact their bodies were prisoners, they had the freedom of their minds.

When you are confined in the prison camp of injury you have no control. People move you around, direct your days and even force their way into dreams. For those who can remember the time when they made decisions, made things happen, the loss of control often causes a panic that is expressed outwardly in various fashions.

Help your loved one have some control, if only over what you may perceive is small and inconsequential. By doing so you may short circuit other problems. You may know best; you may love them very much; you may be afraid to let them choose, but love them enough to let go; let them make a mistake. They'll thank you for it someday.

Monday 38

It is only when we actually begin a difficult task that we find we have the power and talent to carry it off. As long as we sit and think about it, wish for it and stay where we are, nothing happens.

A favorite expression of James Lincoln, the man who built the Lincoln Electric Company was: "You never know what a man can do until he has been given sufficient incentive to strive his utmost to bring out the God given abilities within him." How many Fords and Edisons go to their grave unrecognized the world will never know.
The tragedy is they were never given sufficient incentive or never met a crisis in their lives that brought out their hidden powers."

Somerset Maugham once wrote: "It's a funny thing about life--if you refuse to accept anything but the best, you very often get it." We get what we expect from life. We get from our special family members often what we expect from them, when we expect nothing less than their best effort. We have to in the days, months, and maybe years to come, give them the incentive to do their best and never let them know that we expect or will accept anything less than the best they can do. When we do that we give them the best gift of all. Freedom from us. There's no playing safe. As long as the baseball player keeps one foot on first base he will never go to second. As long as we maintain an environment that is comfortable we stop going forward. If we do only what is required of us, we remain like slaves to the condition. When we do more than is required, only then are we free.

Monday 39

There may be days when you're already hurting, feelings will scream NO MORE! The friends you thought would be there for you, the best friend of your child, the spouse's best buddy, may have all faded from the picture. That hurts. You thought you could count on them; they would say they thought so too, but many just don't or can't deal with the recovery process.

Well I'd be there for them, you think. Maybe you would, maybe not. We never know until we're confronted with something just how we will handle it. Put them and your hurt and resentful feelings aside. Put it over there with all those things you can't do anything about.

Forgive them and their inability to handle the situation. They are only human and have the frailities of humanity. Lean on the power that isn't human for support and sustained strength.

Monday 40

Things happen to all of us caused by external as well as internal forces. Most of our lives are governed by the external. Weather, job, laws, taxes and accidents. Sometimes, however, we find ourselves in much the same predicament as the small game hunter who decided it was now time to go after some big game. His choice of big game was a bear. He must have bear.

Never having hunted for bear, as he wandered around the woods the bear spotted him before he spotted the bear. When the dust settled the hunter lay on his back with the Grizzly sitting astride him, hands folded as if in prayer.

Mustering internal forces the hunter decided it was time for him, with what time he might have left, to make a commitment to God. After doing so he prayed. "Oh God PLEASE let this bear be a Christian." Having asked this he opened his eyes. He beheld the bear, still sitting with paws together saying, "thank you

God for this meal I'm about to receive."

A lack of commitment to God did not cause our hunter to be the bear's dinner, but being prepared for the external forces that could affect his life could have prevented him from being the bear's main course.

As you face the recovery process internally as well as externally, begin to prepare. Read; ask questions; seek your own answers; take offered help and support. Don't let the trauma have YOU for lunch.

Monday 41

If I had to choose among all the people I call my friends the one I count on the most, the one I can tell anything to, the one who has always been there, I'd have to choose Carole. Carole's mother recently died after years of battling with cancer.

During Irma's struggle to win the war time and time again, I tried to remember to send her cards and notes of encouragement. But her will and her desire to be victorious set a wonderful example for me and she gave me far more from being that example than I ever gave her.

The day came when Irma had had enough. There were to be no

more treatments, no more tube feedings, NO MORE. When Irma decided it was time, she met death on her terms and was gone within 24 hours. The will that had kept her alive for her seven year battle, now enabled her to die with the same determination and dignity with which she lived her life.

The power of the human will to live/die is a magnificent power. A power most of us leave forever untapped. You can draw on yours now. Use it as a tool, make it work for you. Use that power, the power within you to be the best you can be.

Monday 42

Our concern must be to live while we're alive...to release our inner selves from the spiritual death that comes with leaving behind a facade designed to conform to the external definitions of who and what we are.

Elizabeth Kubler-Ross

Only when we have braved and gone through the fire of traumatic illness or injury can we read this and truly understand what has been so poignantly said.

Now that we've gotten through, it's even more important that we remember this and don't erect the facade of the injury.

Monday 43

What do they know about what I'm going through? Their child is graduating from high school. Mine never will.
Their child is going off to college.
Mine never will.
Their son is getting married. Mine never will.
Their daughter is having a baby. Mine never will have the opportunity to know that joy.

How did they get so lucky? Their kids weren't perfect, but they're not hurt. Why did it happen to mine?

Accidents, disease, death happens. We weren't singled out. God didn't say - You, You, and You, trouble in your life, bad times ahead, and then sit back arms folded, to watch you struggle. It just doesn't happen that way.

Many will never know the pain you're going through, but then there are many who never had the opportunity to know the years of love, laughter, joy that your loved one brought, just by their presence in your life, even for what now seems like a short time. Many will never marry. Many will never hold a new baby of their own; many will never experience loving or being loved.

Rejoice in the blessing you were allowed to have, if only for a short time. Hold that memory close, and say good-bye to what was. Open your arms and welcome the person that is now.

Monday 44

It seems that each new year brings with it some new psychological "Buzz Words." We've been through "dysfunctional", and "psycho-bable", and one that particularly drives me crazy, "co-dependent". There is a not-so-new but more visible one making the rounds currently. Speakers, authors, many are using the word "Empowerment".

How much more that word says to our psyche. Much more than enable, help, support emPOWERment. Aiding by power, one's own power; especially when s/he may feel s/he has none. What a great word. What a great feeling to give it. The best part of all, one human being can do it. It doesn't take a power company.

One human being. Is it you?

Monday 45

Rehabilitation can be a long process. I'm officially out of therapy but continue to use compensatory strategies daily to help me make it through. I still recheck and second guess myself. What I don't do is let it stop me from doing. I say yes; I will do that. Yes, I can do that, and then sometimes I ask myself, HOW! am I going to do that. HOW! do I get it done.

Many will have to do the same thing. Whether its learning to walk again, using crutches, or a walker. Going out into the world in a wheelchair. We all have to take a step, that first one. A step of faith. And even if the first step is wavering, uneven, unsure, how must we walk? Faith's way.

Monday
46

General H. Norman Schwarzkopf, in his speech at the U.S. Military Academy, spoke on leadership.

One type, he suggested led with competance and did whatever it took to get the awards, pile up the achievements and make their way to the top. They sacrificed character.

He also said he had met many with character but who lacked competence. They were not willing to go that extra step it took to be a leader.

These qualities are important in families and in those people who will direct your rehabilitation or that of your loved one. The fight to regain a life is every bit as important as any war fought anywhere, for any reason.

BRAIN INJURY GLOSSARY

A GLOSSARY OF TERMS AND DEFINITIONS OF INTEREST TO:

FAMILY MEMBERS AND SURVIVORS OF BRAIN INJURY

CASE MANAGERS

INSURANCE REPRESENTATIVES

STAFFS OF HEALTH CARE FACILITIES

STAFF OF GOVERNMENTAL AGENCIES

LOCAL, STATE, REGIONAL, AND NATIONAL
HEAD (BRAIN) INJURY ORGANIZATIONS

Compiled by Staff of
The Institute for Rehabilitation and Research (TIRR)
Traumatic Brain Injury (TBI) Model System Research Program
Texas Medical Center
1333 Moursund Avenue
Houston, TX 77030

November 1990

(Reprinted May, 1991)

Edited by:

L. Don Lehmkuhl, PhD
Manager, TBI Model System Research Program
TIRR
Texas Medical Center
1333 Moursund Avenue
Houston, TX 77030
713-666-7323; FAX 713-668-5210

Please direct any suggestions for revision to Dr. Lehmkuhl

Single copies or bulk quantities of this glossary can be ordered from the National Head Injury Foundation, 1140 Connecticut Avenue, Suite 812, Washington, DC 20036 (202) 296-NHIF.

Acknowledgements:

Prepared with financial assistance from Grant G0087C2016 awarded by the U.S. Department of Education, National Institute on Disability and Rehabilitation Research (NIDRR) to the TIRR Brain Injury Rehabilitation Program, Catherine F. Bontke, MD, Principal Investigator and L. Don Lehmkuhl, PhD, Project Manager.

The assistance of the following TIRR staff members is gratefully acknowledged:

Mary Finn, Research Associate-Database (1987-89)
Linda Thoi, Research Associate-Database (1989-present)
Lani Worthington, Research Associate-Clinical (1987-88)
Rob Stradtner, Research Associate-Clinical (1988-present)
Eileen Lofft (1988-89), Dawn May (1989-90) and Melanie Budnik (1990-present), Secretaries

November 1990
(Reprinted May, 1991)

FORWARD

This glossary was originally compiled for use in discussions with staffs of the five Traumatic Brain Injury (TBI) Model Systems (TIRR in Houston, TX; Santa Clara Valley Medical Center in San Jose, CA; Medical College of Virginia in Richmond, VA; Mount Sinai Medical Center in New York City, NY; and the Rehabilitation Institute of Michigan in Detroit, MI) recently funded by the National Institute on Disability and Rehabilitation Research (NIDRR). These TBI Model Systems were selected to develop and field test a national data set for characterizing persons who have received a traumatic brain injury and in following their progress through acute care, rehabilitation and re-integration into the community. The five TBI Model Systems have been joined by a Rehabilitation Research and Training Center-TBI at the State University of New York in Buffalo, NY, which has been designated to receive and analyze the data collected by the five Model Systems. We soon realized that a glossary of terms compiled for our use would also be of interest to others in the field of Brain Injury. Therefore, early drafts of this glossary were distributed widely to solicit content that will be of widespread use. The terms and definitions have been drawn from a large number of sources. Those which could be identified are listed in the bibliography. No attempt has been made to trace the <u>original</u> source of a definition because many of the sources available to us were too far removed from any original publication of the definition.

As the result of a consensus of leaders in brain injury research assembled at the NIDRR Medical Sciences Project Directors Conference held in Tyson's Corner, VA, October 10-11, 1990, the editor has replaced the term "head injury" with "brain injury" throughout this glossary. This is being done to more accurately reflect the anatomical basis of the problems being addressed. Damage to the "brain" results in dysfunction of the brain which is responsible for the observable disabilities.

We hope that this document, and future refinements of it, will serve as the basis for standardizing terms and definitions in the field of Brain Injury Rehabilitation and for improving communication among health professionals working in this field. Another significant goal is to assist in improving communication between health professionals and other interested parties, such as family members of persons who have survived a brain injury and staff members of insurance carriers or of governmental agencies. A serious attempt has been made to prepare definitions which can be understood by persons not specifically educated in a health profession. Previous drafts have been reviewed and critiqued by family members of patients undergoing rehabilitation, by staff of the National Head Injury Foundation (NHIF) and by members of the Head Injury Interdisciplinary Special Interest Group (ISIG) of the American Congress of Rehabilitation Medicine (ACRM). Your suggestions for improvement in this Glossary are welcome. Address correspondence to:

L. Don Lehmkuhl, PhD
Editor, BRAIN INJURY GLOSSARY
TIRR
1333 Moursund Avenue
Houston, TX 77030

TIRR BRAIN INJURY GLOSSARY

Abnormal — Not normal.

Abscess — A localized collection of pus in a cavity.

Abstract Concept — Refers to a concept that is not easily related to any specific instance and may therefore be difficult to understand. Patients with cognitive deficits usually have difficulty understanding abstract concepts.

Abstract Thinking — A style of thinking in which language is interpreted conceptually. The ability to reason and to solve problems.

Acalculia — The inability to perform simple problems of arithmetic.

Accident — See appended GLOSSARY OF INSURANCE TERMS.

Acuity — Sharpness or quality of a sensation.

Acute — Sharp, severe, having sudden onset, sharp rise and short course.

Acute Care — See Program Type

Acute Rehabilitation Program — Primary emphasis is on the early phase of rehabilitation which usually begins as soon as the patient is medically stable. The program is designed to be comprehensive and based in a medical facility with a typical length of stay of 2-3 months. Treatment is provided by an identifiable team in a designated unit.

Adaptive/Assistive Equipment — A special device which assists in the performance of self-care, work or play/leisure activities or physical exercise.

Adaptive Physical Conditioning — Developing the patient's strengths and ability to overcome a handicapping condition.

Adiadochokinesia — Inability to stop one movement and follow it immediately with movement in the opposite direction.

ADL — Activities of daily living. Routine activities carried out for personal hygiene and health (including bathing, dressing, feeding) and for operating a household.

TIRR BRAIN INJURY GLOSSARY

Advocacy Organization	A group or nonprofit entity which provides resource information, support services and/or educational opportunities for individuals or families in need, and makes those needs known to professional caregivers as well as to the general public.
Affect	The emotional state of an individual at any given time.
Affective Disorders	Mental illnesses characterized mainly by abnormalities in mood. The two principal categories are mania and depression.
Agnosia	Failure to recognize familiar objects although the sensory mechanism is intact. May occur for any sensory modality.
Agraphia	Inability to express thoughts in writing.
Akinetic Mutism	A condition of silent, alert-appearing, immobility that characterizes certain subacute or chronic states of altered consciousness. Sleep-wake cycles have been retained, but no observable evidence for mental activity is evident; spontaneous motor activity is lacking; patient appears to be aware but inactive. Exhibited by patients with high brainstem lesions.
Alert	State of being watchful or ready.
Alexia	Inability to read.
Ambulate	To walk.
Amnesia	Lack of memory about events occurring during a particular period of time.
Aneurysm	A balloon-like deformity in the wall of a blood vessel. The wall weakens as the balloon grows larger, and may eventually burst, causing a hemorrhage.
Anomia	Inability to recall names of objects. Patients with this problem often can speak fluently but have to use other words to describe familiar objects.
Anosmia	Loss of the sense of smell.

TIRR BRAIN INJURY GLOSSARY

Anoxia	A lack of oxygen. Cells of the brain need oxygen to stay alive. When blood flow to the brain is reduced or when oxygen in the blood is too low, brain cells are damaged.
Anterograde Amnesia	Inability to consolidate information about ongoing events. Difficulty with new learning.
Anticoagulation	Process of "thinning the blood." Medication (Heparin, Coumadin) is used to slow down normal blood clotting and thus prevent blood clots from forming.
Anticonvulsant	Medication used to decrease the possibility of a seizure (e.g., Dilantin, Phenobarbitol, Mysoline, Tegretol).
Antidepressants	Medication used to treat depression.
Apallic Syndrome (This is an older, non-specific term. See Persistent Vegetative State)	The behavior that accompanies diffuse bilateral degeneration of the cerebral cortex that sometimes follows anoxic brain injury. It describes patients with absent cortical function but with relatively intact brainstem function.
Apathy	A lack of interest or concern.
Aphasia	Loss of the ability to express oneself and/or to understand language. Caused by damage to brain cells rather than deficits in speech or hearing organs.
Aphasia, Expressive	Inability to find or formulate the words to express oneself even though knowing what one wants to say.
Aphasia, Global	Severely limited residual ability to communicate with others. Includes both expressive and receptive aphasia.
Aphasia, Nonfluent	Characterized by awkward articulation, limited vocabulary, hesitant, slow speech output, restricted use of grammatical forms and a relative preservation of auditory comprehension.
Aphasia, Receptive	Problems in understanding what others attempt to communicate.

TIRR BRAIN INJURY GLOSSARY

Aphasia, Sub-clinical	Refers to evidence of impaired linguistic processing on testing, which is not obvious in casual interactions with the person.
Aphemia	The isolated loss of the ability to articulate words without loss of the ability to write or comprehend spoken language.
Apraxia	Inability to carry out a complex or skilled movement not due to paralysis, sensory changes, or deficiencies in understanding.
Apraxia, Constructional	Inability to assemble, build, draw, or copy accurately; not due to apraxia of single movements.
Apraxia, Ideomotor	Deficit in the execution of a movement due to inability to access the instructions to muscles stored by previous motor experience.
Arousal	Being awake. Primitive state of alertness managed by the reticular activating system (extending from medulla to the thalamus in the core of the brainstem) activating the cortex. Cognition is not possible without some degree of arousal.
Art Therapy	Use of art techniques such as painting, crafts and group activities to develop motor skills, perceptual abilities and self-esteem.
Arterial Line	A very thin tube (catheter) inserted into an artery to allow direct measurement of the blood pressure, the oxygen and carbon dioxide concentrations in arterial blood.
Arterio-venous Malformation-AVM	A "tangle" of blood vessels present from birth which may be prone to bleeding.
Articulation	Movement of the lips, tongue, teeth and palate into specific patterns for purposes of speech. Also, a movable joint.
Aspiration	When fluid or food enters the lungs through the wind pipe. Can cause a lung infection or pneumonia.
Associated Reaction	A non-purposeful movement that accompanies another movement (e.g., patient's arm may bend involuntarily when the patient yawns).

TIRR BRAIN INJURY GLOSSARY

Astereognosia	Inability to recognize things by touch.
Ataxia	A problem of muscle coordination not due to apraxia, weakness, rigidity, spasticity or sensory loss. Caused by lesion of the cerebellum or basal ganglia. Can interfere with a person's ability to walk, talk, eat, and to perform other self care tasks.
Atrophy	A wasting away or decrease in size of a cell, tissue, organ, or part of the body caused by lack of nourishment or loss of nerve supply.
Attention, Alternating	Is the ability to move attention appropriately from one selective focus to another. It is an aspect of control, but one that requires capacity.
Attention/ Concentration	The ability to focus on a given task or set of stimuli for an appropriate period of time.
Attention/ Concentration, Distractibility	Refers to the patient's inability to sustain attention because of competing internal or external stimuli. Typically, the person with a brain injury has decreased ability to inhibit inappropriate responses. For example, a restrained patient may focus more on his arm restraint than on a task presented by a therapist; a patient asked to complete arithmetic problems may focus more on construction work taking place outside.
Attention/ Concentration, Arousal	The ability to respond consistently to sensory stimulation by eye opening, localizing, and tracking with head or eye movement. To assess a comatose patient's level of arousal one might determine if the patient brushes away pinching fingers; or, if the head turns to a voice or noise.
Attention/ Concentration, Length	Refers to the amount of time a patient is able to focus on a given task. Complexity of task and patient fatigability will affect length of attention.
Attention, Divided	Refers to an attentional task where the performer must attend to two or more inputs or activities at the same time.

TIRR BRAIN INJURY GLOSSARY

Attention, Selective	Term refers to selection of a particular train of thought rather than others as the focus of attention.
Attention, Sustained	Refers to a person's ability to work on a particular task or train of thought over an extended period of time.
Attention Span	The length of time one is able to concentrate on a task at hand.
Attention to Task	Ability to focus on a given activity.
Audiologist	One who evaluates hearing defects and who aids in the rehabilitation of those who have such defects.
Augmentative and Alternative Communication	An area of speech-language pathology clinical practice in which attempts are made to compensate (either temporarily or permanently) for severe expressive communication disorders.
Automatic Speech	Words said without much thinking on the part of the speaker. These may include songs, numbers, and social communication; or, can be items previously learned through memorization. Spontaneous swearing by individuals who did not do so before their injury is another example.
Awareness	Conscious of stimulation, arising from within or from outside the person.
Awareness, Deficit	The patient's inability to recognize the problems caused by impaired brain function.
Awareness, Emergent	Problem when occurring patients must first be aware that a problem exists.
Awareness, Level Of	Rating by a qualified observer of the degree to which a patient is perceiving internal and external stimuli.
Balance	The ability to use appropriate righting and equilibrium reactions to maintain an upright position. It is usually tested in sitting and standing positions.
Behavior	The total collection of actions and reactions exhibited by a person.
Benefits	See appended GLOSSARY OF INSURANCE TERMS.

TIRR BRAIN INJURY GLOSSARY

Behavior Disorders — See Program Type

Bilateral — Pertaining to both right and left sides.

Biofeedback — A process in which information not ordinarily perceived (such as heart rate, skin temperature or electrical activity of muscles) is recorded from a person and then relayed back instantaneously as a signal so that the individual becomes aware of any alteration in the recorded activity.

Blind — Describes a condition in which a person has lost vision for ordinary life purposes. Generally, anyone with less than 10% of normal vision would be regarded as legally blind.

Brain Death — A state in which all functions of the brain (cortical, subcortical, and brainstem) are permanently lost.

Brain Injury, Closed — Occurs when the head collides with another object (for example the windshield of a car) and brain tissue is damaged, not by the presence of a foreign object within the brain, but by violent smashing, stretching, and twisting, of brain tissue. Closed head injuries typically cause diffuse tissue damage that results in disabilities which are generalized and highly variable.

Brain Injury, Mild — A patient with a mild traumatic brain injury is a person who has had a traumatically-induced physiological disruption of cerebral function, as manifested by **at least** one of the following: 1) any period of loss of consciousness, 2) any loss of memory for events immediately before or after the accident (retrograde or anterograde amnesia); any alteration in mental state at the time of the accident (e.g. feeling dazed, disoriented, or confused), even in the absence of loss of consciousness or amnesia; 4) physical symptoms which are potentially brain related (e.g. nausea, vomiting, dizziness, headache, tinnitus, blurred vision, other sensory loss such as taste or smell, or extended periods of fatigue and lethargy); 5) development of post-traumatic cognitive deficits (e.g. attention, concentration, memory, language, perception, etc.), which cannot be completely accounted for by emotional state; but where the severity of the injury does not exceed the following: a) loss of consciousness of approximately 30 minutes or less; b) after 30 minutes, an initial Glasgow Coma Scale of 13-15; c) Post Traumatic Amnesia not greater than 24 hours.

Brain Injury, Moderate — A Glasgow Coma Score of 9 to 12 at the time of admission. Two-thirds of moderately-injured persons remain moderately-disabled or severely-disabled three months post injury.

Brain Injury, Penetrating — Occurs when an object (for example a bullet or an ice pick) fractures the skull, enters the brain and rips the soft brain tissue in its path. Penetrating injuries tend to damage relatively localized areas of the brain which result in fairly discrete and predictable disabilities.

Brain Injury, Severe — Severe injury is one that produces at least 6 hours of coma; Glasgow Coma Score of 8 or less within the first 24 hours.

Brain Injury, Traumatic — Damage to living brain tissue caused by an external, mechanical force. It is usually characterized by a period of altered consciousness (amnesia or coma) that can be very brief (minutes) or very long (months/indefinitely). The resulting tissue damage impairs an individual's mental, and/or psychosocial abilities. Also called traumatic brain injury (TBI).

Brain Plasticity — The ability for structure and functions to be molded and shaped according to the environmental demands; diminishes with maturation.

Brain Scan — An imaging technique in which a radioactive dye is injected into the blood stream and then pictures of the brain are taken to detect tumors, hemorrhages, blood clots, abscesses or abnormal anatomy.

Brainstem — The lower extension of the brain where it connects to the spinal cord. Neurological functions located in the brainstem include those necessary for survival (breathing, heart rate) and for arousal (being awake and alert).

Capacity, Mental	Capacity refers to the amount of information or mental processing a person can attend to within a given time.
Case Management	Facilitating the access of a patient to appropriate rehabilitation and support programs, and coordination of the delivery of services. This role may involve liaison with various professionals and agencies, advocacy on behalf of the patient, and arranging for purchase of services where no appropriate programs are available.
Catheter	A flexible tube for withdrawing fluids from, or introducing fluids into, a cavity of the body. Frequently used to drain the urinary bladder (Foley catheter).
Cerebellum	The portion of the brain (located at the back) which helps coordinate movement. Damage may result in ataxia.
Cerebral Angiography	A medical test involving injection of dye into an artery so that the vascular system of the brain can be studied through an x-ray; can detect aneurysms, tumors, or circulation problems.
Cerebral Compression	The brain substance is pushed aside and compressed by the presence of a brain tumor, aneurysm, swelling or hematoma.
Cerebral Infarct	When the blood supply is reduced below a critical level and the brain tissue in that region dies.
Cerebrospinal Fluid	Liquid (CSF) which fills the ventricles of the brain and surrounds the brain and spinal cord.
Chemically Dependent	Drug dependent.
Chemotherapy	The treatment of a condition by the systematic administration of chemical compounds.
Chest tubes	Tubes inserted into the patient's chest between the lung and ribs to allow fluid

	and air to drain from the area surrounding the lungs. Removing this fluid and air from around the lungs allows them to more fully expand.
Chronic	Marked by long duration or frequent recurrence.
Chronic Care	Long-term care for those individuals who require nursing care; a maintenance program to prevent deterioration of skills, and to provide recreational and social opportunities in a structured environment. Emphasis is on improving the quality of life, and expectations regarding improvements in abilities are limited.
Circumlocution	Use of other words to describe a specific word or idea which cannot be remembered.
Claim	See appended GLOSSARY OF INSURANCE TERMS.
Cleft Lip	Specific congenital disability involving lip and gum. The term hare lip is anatomically incorrect and stigmatizing.
Clonus	A sustained series of rhythmic jerks following quick stretch of a muscle.
Closed Head Injury	See Brain Injury, Closed.
Congenital Disability	A disability that has existed since birth but is not necessarily hereditary. The term birth defect is inappropriate.
Cognition	The conscious process of knowing or being aware of thoughts or perceptions, including understanding and reasoning.
Cognitive Rehabilitation	Therapy programs which aid persons surviving brain injury in the management of specific problems in thinking and perception. Skills are practiced and strategies are taught to help improve function and/or compensate for remaining deficits.
Coinsurance	See appended GLOSSARY OF INSURANCE TERMS.
Coma	A state of unconsciousness from which the patient cannot be aroused, even by powerful stimulation.

TIRR BRAIN INJURY GLOSSARY

Coma Management Program	See Program Type.
Coma Vigil (See Persistent Vegetative State)	A patient who neither responds to commands nor moves despite the appearance of cognitive readiness and sustained wakefulness.
Commensurate Wage	A wage paid to a handicapped worker which is comparable to wages paid to a nonhandicapped worker in the vicinity, performing similar work at a specific quality level, with the quantity factor being the main variable.
Communicative Disorder	An impairment in the ability to 1) receive and/or process a symbol system, 2) represent concepts or symbol systems, and/or 3) transmit and use symbol systems. The impairment is observed in disorders of hearing, language, and/or speech processes.
Community Alter-natives	Agencies, outside an institutional setting, which provide care, support, and/or services to handicapped individuals.
Community - Based Programs	Programs for handicapped which are located in a community environment, as opposed to an institutional setting.
Community Resources	Public or private agencies, schools, or programs offering service to people in the field of social services. They are usually funded by governmental bodies, community drives, donations, and fees.
Community Skills	Those abilities needed to function independently in the community. They may include: telephone skills, money management, pedestrian skills, meal planning and cooking, use of public transportation.
Competitive Bid	An agreement to perform specified work under specified conditions and for a specified price which has been determined through the use of the same cost estimating procedures as those of competitive private industrial concerns.
Comprehension	Understanding of spoken, written, or gestural communication.

TIRR BRAIN INJURY GLOSSARY

Concentration	Maintaining attention on a task over a period of time; remaining attentive and not easily diverted.
Concrete Thinking	A style of thinking in which the individual sees each situation as unique and is unable to generalize from the similarities between situations. Thinking in which language is interpreted literally.
Concussion	The common result of a blow to the head usually causing unconsciousness, either temporary or prolonged. Physiologic and/or anatomic disruption of connections between some nerve cells in the brain may occur.
Confabulation	Verbalizations about people, places, and events with no basis in reality. The patient appears to "fill in" gaps in memory with plausible facts.
Confusion	A state in which a person is bewildered, perplexed, or unable to self-orient.
Conjugate Movement	Both eyes move simultaneously in the same direction. Convergence of the eyes toward the midline (crossed eyes) is a disconjugate movement.
Consciousness	The state of awareness of the self and the environment.
Consumer	An individual who, by reason of disability, is eligible for, may require, has received, or is recipient of some kind of human service, including medical, rehabilitation, housing, transportation, etc.
Continent	The ability to control urination and bowel movements.
Contractures	Loss of range of motion in a joint due to abnormal shortening of soft tissues.
Contralateral	Opposite side.
Control of Attention	Control refers to a person's ability to guide the selective process by directing and organizing whatever attentional capacity he or she has.
Contusion	A bruise. The result of a blow to the head which bruises the brain.
Convergence	Movement of two eyeballs inward to focus on

an object moved closer. The nearer the object, the greater is the degree of convergence necessary to maintain single vision.

Coping Skills — The ability to deal with problems and difficulties by attempting to overcome them or accept them.

Core Therapies — Basic therapy services provided by professionals on a brain injury rehabilitation unit. Usually refers to nursing, physical therapy, occupational therapy, speech-language pathology, neuropsychology, social work and therapeutic recreation.

Cortical Blindness — Loss of vision resulting from a lesion of the primary visual areas of the occipital lobe. Light reflex is preserved.

Contrecoup — Bruising of brain tissue on the side opposite where the blow was struck.

Coup Damage — Damage to the brain at the point of impact.

CT Scan/ Computerized Axial Tomography — A series of X-rays taken at different levels of the brain that allows the direct visualization of intracranial structures. A scan is often taken soon after the injury to help decide if surgery is needed. The scan may be repeated later to see how the brain is recovering.

Cue — A signal or direction used to assist a person in performing an activity (telling a person the initial of your first name serves as a cue when he cannot remember your name).

Dance/Movement Therapy — The use of movement to music as a process which enhances, facilitates and integrates physical, cognitive and psychosocial function.

Day Care — A service provided during ordinary working hours for the patient who requires supervision, including assistance with medication, meal preparation, dressing or moving about. However, the family returns the patient to their residence and assumes responsibility for care during the evenings and at night.

TIRR BRAIN INJURY GLOSSARY

Day Treatment Program — See Program Type

Deaf — Deafness refers to a profound degree of hearing loss that prevents understanding speech through the ear.

Decerebrate Posture (Decerebrate Rigidity) — Exaggerated posture of extension as a result of a lesion to the prepontine area of the brainstem, and is rarely seen fully developed in humans. In reporting, it is preferable to describe the posture seen.

Decorticate Posture (Decorticate Rigidity) — Exaggerated posture of upper extremity flexion and lower extremity extension as a result of a lesion to the mesencephalon or above. In reporting, it is preferable to describe the posture seen.

Decubitus — Pressure area, bed sore, skin opening, skin breakdown. A discolored or open area of skin damage caused by pressure. Common areas most prone to breakdown are buttocks or backside, hips, shoulder blades, heels, ankles and elbows.

Deep Vein Thrombosis (DVT) — A blood clot in a vein, located deep from the skin, most commonly seen in the calf or thigh. Veins lying just beneath the skin are called superficial veins.

Deficit — A deficiency in amount or quality of functioning.

Deinstitutionalization — A concept which has three interrelated processes: 1) avoiding placement in a public institution by developing, finding, and using alternative community methods of care and training; 2) return to the community of those residents who can function appropriately and who can benefit from community-based rehabilitation and training programs; and 3) establishment and maintenance of a responsible institutional environment which protects the human and civil rights of handicapped individuals and which contributes to the appropriate and prompt return of the individual to the community.

Developmental Disability — Any mental and/or physical disability that has an onset before age 22 and may continue indefinitely. It can limit major life activities. Term includes individuals with mental retardation, cerebral palsy, autism, epilepsy (and other seizure disorders), sensory impairments, congenital disabilities, traumatic accidents, or conditions caused by disease (e.g. polio, muscular dystrophy).

Diaschisis — A theoretical state following brain injury in which healthy areas connected to the damaged area show a temporary loss of function.

Diffuse Axonal Injury (DAI) — A shearing injury of large nerve fibers (axons covered with myelin) in many areas of the brain. It appears to be one of the two primary lesions of brain injury, the other being stretching or shearing of blood vessels from the same forces, producing hemorrhage.

Diffuse Brain Injury — Injury to cells in many areas of the brain rather than in one specific location due to the brain moving about and tissue being torn, stretched, and bruised.

Diplopia — Seeing two images of a single object; double vision.

Disability — Any restriction or lack of ability, resulting from an impairment, to perform an everyday activity in the manner or within the range considered normal for a person of the same age, culture, and education.

Disadvantaged Individual — Any individual constrained by reason of physical or mental disability, youth, advanced age, low educational attainment, ethnic or cultural factors, prison or delinquency records, or any other condition, especially in association with poverty.

Discrimination, Sensory — A process requiring differentiation of two or more stimuli.

Discrimination, Auditory — The ability to differentiate and recognize sounds. This involves distinguishing between words, noises, and sounds that might be similar. A patient with poor auditory discrimination might answer the phone in his room although the actual ringing came from an alarm clock.

Discrimination, Tactile	The ability to identify and distinguish between objects and stimuli solely through touch. This involves the ability to ascertain shape, size, and texture. For example, patients with impaired tactile discrimination might not be able to distinguish between a quarter and a dime in their pocket.
Discrimination, Visual	Involves the differentiation of items using sight. An individual with impaired visual discrimination may not be able to distinguish between a red and green light while driving or may have difficulty distinguishing between the letter "E" and the letter "F".
Disinhibition	Inability to suppress (inhibit) impulsive behavior and emotions.
Disorientation	Not knowing where you are, who you are, or the current date. Health professionals often speak of a normal person as being oriented "times three" which refers to person, place and time.
Disposition	Plans for where the person will live after discharge from the hospital and who will be able to help that individual.
Distal	Far from the point of attachment.
Doll's Eye Maneuver	The eyes appear to move in the direction opposite to the motion of the head, when the head is gently rotated.
Dorsiflexion	When applied to the ankle, the ability to bend at the ankle, moving the front of the foot upward.
Down Syndrome	A form of mental retardation caused by improper chromosomal division during fetal development.
Dysarthria	Difficulty in forming words or speaking them because of weakness of muscles used in speaking. Speech is characterized by slurred, imprecise articulation. Tongue movements are usually labored and the rate of speaking may be very slow. Voice quality may be abnormal, usually excessively nasal; volume may be weak;

	drooling may occur. Dysarthria may accompany aphasia or occur alone.
Dysmetria	Inability to stop a movement at the desired point; also known as past-pointing.
Dysphagia	A swallowing disorder characterized by difficulty in oral preparation for the swallow, or in moving material from the mouth to the stomach. This definition also includes problems in positioning food in the mouth.
Echolalia	Imitation of sounds or words without comprehension. Is a normal stage of language development in infants, but is abnormal in adults.
Edema	Collection of fluid in the tissue causing swelling.
Education Program	See Program Type
EEG/Electro-encephalogram	A procedure that uses electrodes on the scalp to record electrical activity of the brain. Used for detection of epilepsy, coma, and death.
ECG/EKG Electro-cardiogram	Usually three small, round electrode pads located on the patient's chest to monitor heart rate and rhythm. These are connected to a monitor and used routinely in the intensive care unit.
EMG/Electromyo-graphy	An insertion of needle electrodes into muscles to study the electrical activity of muscle and nerve fibers. It may be somewhat painful to the patient. Helps diagnose partial denervation.
Embolism	The sudden blocking of an artery or a vein by a blood clot, bubble of air, deposit of oil or fat, or small mass of cells deposited by the blood flow.
Emotional Lability	Exhibiting rapid and drastic changes in emotional state (laughing, crying, anger) without apparent reason.
Employment Program	See Program Type
Encephalography	Non-invasive use of ultrasound waves to record echoes from brain tissue. Used to

detect hematoma, tumor, or ventricle problems.

Endotracheal Tube — A tube that serves as an artificial airway and is inserted through the patient's mouth or nose. It passes through the throat and into the air passages to help breathing. To do this it must also pass through the patient's vocal cords. The patient will be unable to speak as long as the endotracheal tube is in place. It is this tube that connects the respirator to the patient.

Engram — A lasting mark or trace. The term is applied to the bioelectrical trace associated with storage of a memory in the nervous system.

Environmental Working Conditions — Those physical surroundings of job/worker situations which make specific demands upon a worker's physical capacity.

Equilibrium — Normal balance reactions and postures.

Error Correction — Should follow error recognition and refers to the ability to replace an inappropriate response with an appropriate one.

Error Recognition — Refers to a patient's awareness that a response is inappropriate for a task. The patient may simply state, for example, "I know this is wrong", or show a confused, quizzical look after making an inappropriate response.

Evaluation Program — Process of assessment according to a defined set of criteria.

Evaluation In A Workshop Setting — A process through which the client's work potential is assessed in a controlled area using simulated or actual job tasks to assess ability to relate to demands of the work environment and perform adequately. Has the following characteristics: 1) client may or may not be paid; 2) client is exposed to tasks on which performance can be assessed; 3) client's performance is supervised and evaluated in coordination with the evaluation staff; and 4) existence of established evaluation program.

Evaluation In A Vocational Training Setting — An evaluation which has the following characteristics: 1) the client is not paid; 2) the existence of an established vocational training program; 3) primarily for the benefit of the client; 4) client's performance supervised and evaluated by the instructional staff in coordination with evaluation staff; and 5) does not necessarily result in entry by the client into that training program.

Evaluation On-The-Job — Contains at least these characteristics: 1) the client is not necessarily paid; 2) it is primarily for the client's benefit; 3) it will not necessarily result in employment; 4) the employer does not experience any immediate gain; 5) the client does not displace or fill any vacant worker slots; and 6) the client's performance is supervised and evaluated by the employer and/or the evaluation staff. The client is given the opportunity to experience, in various degrees of participation, the specific requirements necessary to do the specific job in an actual job setting.

Evaluation Program — Comprehensive assessment of the problems and capabilities of an individual complete with recommendations for dealing with the problems.

Evaluation - Tools Of — All of the means and media with which the evaluator and the client carry out vocational evaluation.

Evoked Potential — Registration of the electrical response of brain cells as detected by electrodes placed on the surface of the head at various places. The evoked potential, unlike the waves on an EEG, is elicited by a specific stimulus applied to the visual, auditory or other sensory receptors of the body. Evoked potentials are used to diagnose a wide variety of central nervous system disorders.

Evoked Responses, Brainstem — Auditory brain stem responses provoked by discreet sounds delivered to the ears through headphones. These sound waves are converted to nerve impulses by receptors in the ear. A machine is used to test whether the brainstem has received the signals. The quality of the brainstem's response in a comatose patient is thought to be an important indicator of the degree and site of brain injury. Because this test requires very specialized and expensive equipment, it is not available in all hospitals. A more common test is the EEG.

Executive Functions	Planning, prioritizing, sequencing, self-monitoring, self-correcting, inhibiting, initiating, controlling or altering behavior.
Extended Care Facility	A residential facility for the patient who requires 24-hour nursing care (IV, intramuscular injections, special feeding tubes, skin care, oxygen) or rehabilitative therapy, such as physical therapy, occupational therapy, or speech therapy on a less intensive basis than as an inpatient in a comprehensive rehabilitation center. An extended care facility is usually a short-term alternative (2-3 months) prior to placement at home (with outpatient therapy) or in a nursing home.
Extremity	Arm or leg.
Eye Tape	Tape used to close the eyes of a patient who has lost the ability to blink. To protect the eyes and to prevent them from drying out, eye drops may be put into the eyes and the eye tapes may be used to close them.
Figure-Ground	The differentiation between the foreground and the background of a scene; this refers to all sensory systems, including vision, hearing, touch.
Fixation, Visual	A pause of the line of sight on something of interest in the visual world.
Flaccid	Lacking normal muscle tone; limp.
Flexion	Bending a joint.
Fluently	Effortlessly smooth and rapid speech.
Focal	Restricted to one region (as opposed to diffuse).
Focus, Eye	Can imply: 1) convergence of the two eyes, 2) accommodation of the lenses of the two eyes, 3) tracking something by moving the eyes, 4) attending to something. Because the term has several meanings its use should perhaps be avoided.

TIRR BRAIN INJURY GLOSSARY

Foley Catheter — This is a tube inserted into the urinary bladder for drainage of urine. The urine drains through the tube and collects into a plastic bag.

Follow-Up — Supportive assistance during the initial stage of a new program of job placement and which may determine to what degree the past and present program are adequate to meet client needs and/or ascertain the readiness of clients to benefit from new programs.

Follow-Up Information — Data collected after services have been provided.

Frontal Lobe — Front part of the brain; involved in planning, organizing, problem solving, selective attention, personality and a variety of "higher cognitive functions."

Frustration Tolerance — The ability to persist in completing a task despite apparent difficulty. Individuals with a poor frustration tolerance will often refuse to complete tasks which are the least bit difficult. Angry behavior, such as yelling or throwing things while attempting a task is also indicative of poor frustration tolerance.

Functional Ability — Capacity for performing an act that results in a practical end result.

Functional Inde-pendence — The capacity of a person to take care of his own activities of daily living without the help of another person.

Functional Limitations — Restrictions of physical or mental functions which hinder an individual's ability to take care of one's affairs.

Functional Outcome, Optimal — The highest functional level an individual can realize in consideration of social limitations.

Functional Outcomes — Activities in which a person is capable of engaging on a regular basis and which require the use of time, strength, or faculties.

Gainful Occupation — Includes employment in the competitive labor market, practice of a profession, farm or family work (including work for which payment is in kind rather than in cash), sheltered employment, work activity (to the extent that there is net pay), and home industries or other homebound work.

Gait Training — Instruction in walking, with or without equipment; also called "ambulation training."

GI Tube — A tube inserted through a surgical opening into the stomach. It is used to introduce liquids, food, or medication into the stomach when the patient is unable to take these substances by mouth.

Glasgow Coma Scale — A standardized system used to assess the degree of brain impairment and to identify the seriousness of injury in relation to outcome. The system involves three determinants: eye opening, verbal responses and motor response - all of which are evaluated independently according to a numerical value that indicates the level of consciousness and degree of dysfunction. Scores run from a high of 15 to a low of 3. Persons are considered to have experienced a 'mild brain' injury when their score is 13 to 15. A score of 9 to 12 is considered to reflect a 'moderate' brain injury and a score of 8 or less reflects a 'severe' brain injury.

Glasgow Outcome Scale — A system for classifying the outcome of persons who survive. The categories range from 'Good Recovery' in which the patient appears to regain the pre-injury level of social and career activity (even if there are some minor residual abnormal neurological signs); 'Moderate Disability' in which the patient does not regain the former level of activity but is completely independent with respect to the activities of daily living; 'Severe Disability' is defined as a state wherein the conscious, communicating patient is still dependent on the help of others. The original scale had five outcome categories, the newest scale has eight outcome categories. This scale relates to functional independence and not residual deficits.

Habilitation — Process of providing specific learning experiences for those handicapped individuals who have been isolated from such experiences so they can become aware of and develop their abilities and potentials.

Halo	A metal ring used for patients with spinal cord injuries which encircles the patient's head to allow for proper alignment of the neck and spinal column. It is important that the patient with a broken spine remain still in order to prevent further injury to the spinal cord.
Handicap	A disadvantage for a given individual, resulting from an impairment or a disability that limits or prevents the fulfillment of a role that is normal, depending on age, sex, and social and cultural factors, for the individual.
Handicapped Person	Any individual who has a physical or mental disability which, for that individual, constitutes or results in a substantial handicap to employment.
Hard of Hearing	Mild to moderate hearing loss that may or may not be corrected with amplification.
Head Injury	See Brain Injury.
Health Insurance	See appended GLOSSARY OF INSURANCE TERMS.
Hearing Impaired	Generic term preferred by some individuals to refer to any degree of hearing loss--from mild to profound. It includes both hard of hearing and deaf.
Hematoma	The collection of blood in tissues or a space following rupture of a blood vessel.
Regarding Brain:	Epidural - Outside the brain and its fibrous covering, but under the skull. Subdural - Between the brain and its fibrous covering. Intracerebral - In the brain tissue.
Hemianopsia	Visual field cut. Blindness for one half of the field of vision. This is not the right or left eye, but the right or left half of vision in each eye.
Hemiplegia	Paralysis of one side of the body as a result of injury to neurons carrying signals to muscles from the motor areas of the brain.

TIRR BRAIN INJURY GLOSSARY

Hemiparesis — Weakness of one side of the body.

Hemorrhage — Bleeding that occurs following damage to blood vessels. Bleeding may occur within the brain when blood vessels in the brain are damaged. (See hematoma).

High Level Thought Processes — Includes conversion thinking, deductive and inductive reasoning, divergent thinking, and high level problem-solving, including comprehension of a problem, formulation of several alternative solutions based on past experiences or long-term memory, generation of a solution and evaluation of a solution. This differs from organization in that high level thought processes involve the use of multiple strategies.

Homecare Program — See Program Type

Human Services — Activities provided to people to enable them to deal with their personal environment in such a way that they can gain control over their own destinies and exercise freedom of choice in their lives.

Human Services Delivery System — The organizational structure by which necessary activities are provided to those people who need them and includes health care, education, income maintenance, and manpower services.

Hydrocephalus — Enlargement of fluid-filled cavities in the brain, not due to brain atrophy.

ICD — See International Classification of Disease.

ICP — See Intracranial Pressure.

ICU — See Intensive Care Unit.

Impairment — Reduced capacity for functioning. This term may be used in describing the reduction in functions of a single muscle, or organ; or, reduced capacity for social and family relations, independent living or enjoyment of life as the result of some event or illness.

Imperception — Refers to a failure to perceive stimulation on one side of the body when both sides are being stimulated simultaneously (double simultaneous stimulation). It is not due to a primary sensory deficit such as deafness or blindness but appears to be an attentional deficit. It is less severe than "neglect" and may occur in a patient recovering from neglect.

Impulse Control — Refers to the patient's ability to withhold inappropriate verbal or motor responses while completing a task. Patients who act or speak without first considering the consequences are viewed as having poor impulse control.

Income Maintenance Service — Services related to the economic support of persons; welfare and social security are two such services.

Incontinent — Inability to control bowel and bladder functions. Many people who are incontinent can become continent with training.

Incoordination — A problem with coordination of movement of parts of the body, resulting from dysfunction of the nervous system rather than weakness of muscles.

Independent — The ability to perform a task without assistance or supervision.

Independent Living Program — See Program Type

Individual Case Record — Evaluation of the case includes all information obtained about the client prior to, during, and in follow-up. Includes referral information, social and work history, medical information, referral questions, program goals and plans, services to be provided, signed reports and notations related to performance and progress during the evaluation, notes from case conferences, the termination decision, and final report of findings and recommendations.

Individual Program Plan — See client plan.

Industrial Standards — Actual worker requirements from industry based on the expectations of the employer in terms of quality, quantity, and work behaviors.

Inflexible — Inability to adjust to changes.

Initiative	Refers to the individual's ability to begin a series of behaviors directed toward a goal.
Insight Regarding Impairment	The extent to which an individual accurately judges one's own strengths and weaknesses; also called metacognition. A patient's ability in this area may be judged on the basis of actions or statements regarding intended actions. Patients with brain injuries often overestimate their strengths and underestimate their limitations. For example, a patient with right hemisphere damage may attempt to drive a car while out on pass and get involved in a serious accident. A patient with two broken legs in casts may state that he can't walk because he's "too tired."
Insured	See appended GLOSSARY OF INSURANCE TERMS.
Intake	Those activities which result in an individual's entry into the agency and the action taken to finalize arrangements (i.e. funding, housing, programming) necessary for such entry.
Intellect	Pertains to many of the higher functions of the brain.
Intelligence Quotient	It is a measure of general intelligence obtained by testing. It consists of either a ratio of mental age to chronological age or a score of deviation from an expected test performance by age.
Intensive Care Unit	Hospital unit that utilizes highly sophisticated equipment and specially trained nurses to care for patients who are in such serious condition that they must be continuously monitored.
Intensive Rehabilitation	An active, multidisciplinary rehabilitation program provided for several hours daily, using a team approach. Focus is usually on skill development, rather than on treatment of specific deficits.
Intercerebral	Between the cerebral hemispheres.
Interdisciplinary Approach	A method of diagnosis, evaluation, and individual program planning in which two or more specialists, such as medical doctors,

psychologists, recreational therapists, social workers, etc., participate as a team, contributing their skills, competencies, insights, and perspectives to focus on identifying the developmental needs of the handicapped person and on devising ways to meet those needs.

Intermittent Catheterization Program (ICP) — Bladder training program where a catheter is inserted to empty the bladder at regular time intervals.

International Classification of Disease (ICD-9) — A three digit "N" code used to indicate the pathological nature of an injury. The ninth revision of this classification (ICD-9) has been in use for several years. Unfortunately, the term "brain injury" does not appear as a category. There are ten rubrics which cover most brain/head injuries. The ICD is less useful than desired because rubrics are not mutually exclusive. Differences occur in coding from one institution to another. A new version, ICD-10, is under preparation.

Interpersonal Skills — The ability to relate to others in a socially appropriate, meaningful way.

Interview — Communication between two or more persons used for such purposes as diagnosis, education, therapy or just to gain information. Though some interviews are primarily to obtain information and some primarily to give help, most involve a combination of the two.

Intracranial Pressure (ICP) — Cerebro-spinal fluid (CSF) pressure measured from a needle or bolt introduced into the CSF space surrounding the brain. It reflects the pressure inside of the skull.

Intracranial Pressure Monitor — An ICP monitor. A monitoring device to determine the pressure within the brain. It consists of a small tube (catheter) attached to the patient at the skull by either a ventriculostomy, subarachnoid bolt, or screw and is then connected to a transducer, which registers the pressure.

Intracranial Insults — Something that causes injury to the brain. Includes hematomas (intraparenchymal and extraparenchymal; immediate or delayed)

	elevations of intracranial pressure (ICP), brain swelling, edema, and vasospasm.
Intravenous (IV)	Tubing inserted into a vein through which fluids and medications can be given.
Intravenous Board	A simple wooden or plastic board usually attached with tape to the patient's forearm. It prevents bending and dislocation of the intravenous, or arterial lines.
Ipsilateral	Same side of the body.
Ischemia	A severe reduction in the supply of blood to body tissues.
IV	See Intravenous.
Jargon	Spoken language that has a normal rate and rhythm but is full of nonsense words.
Jejunostomy Tube (J Tube)	A type of feeding tube surgically inserted into the small intestine.
Job Analysis	Involves the systematic study of an occupation in terms of what the worker does in relation to data, people, and things; the methods and techniques employed, the machines, tools, equipment, and work aids used; the materials, products, subject matter or services which result, and the traits required of the worker.
Job Bank	A computerized system, developed by the Department of Labor, which maintains an up-to-date listing of job vacancies available through the State Employment Service.
Job Clusters (Work Families, Job Families)	Related occupations grouped on the basis of similar job requirements, such as specific duties on the job, materials and equipment used, skill and knowledge, and worker characteristics required.
Job Development Specialist	Individual who contacts community businesses and industries for the purpose of placing handicapped clients in competitive employment or on-the-job training stations. Includes analyzing the client's capabilities and consulting with the client's counselor, the facility, and the client in recommending the client for a specific job. May also involve provision

of follow-up services relative to the client's on-the-job performance.

Job Exploration — A process whereby an individual is exposed to work experience and occupational information intended to increase ones knowledge of the world of work.

Job Families — See Job Clusters.

Job Samples — See Work Samples.

Job Seeking Skills — Those skills that enable a person to seek out job vacancies and apply for them. Includes knowledge of where to find information about job openings, how to fill out an application, how to take employment tests, how to handle a job interview.

Job Task — Is an actual single work activity that is taken in its entirety, without any changes, directly from a specific job.

Job Tryout — Contains at least the following characteristics: 1) wages paid to the client; 2) primarily for the employer's benefit; 3) the client is an employee; and 4) the setting is controlled by the employer. It is in actuality a placement used with the understanding that the client may not succeed and will be helped further if he does not. The success or failure provides the evaluator and client with additional information to make specific employment decisions.

Judgement — Process of forming an opinion, based upon an evaluation of the situation at hand in comparison with personal values, preferences and insights. The ability to make appropriate decisions.

Judgement of Safety — The extent to which an individual can correctly judge the dangers and risks in a variety of situations. A patient with poor judgement may smoke in bed late at night, touch a red hot stove burner, or show extreme friendliness to complete strangers. Brain-injured persons with poor insight regarding their impairments are also likely to show poor judgement of safety.

TIRR BRAIN INJURY GLOSSARY

Kinesthesia	The sensory awareness of body parts as they move (see position sense and proprioception).
Lability	State of having notable shifts in emotional state (e.g., uncontrolled laughing or crying).
Laceration	A ragged tear.
Language	The system used to communicate thoughts through symbols.
Latency of Response/ Delay	The amount of time it takes a person to respond after the stimulus has been presented.
Leg Bag	A small, thick plastic bag that can be tied to the leg and collects urine. It is connected by tubing to a catheter inserted into the urinary bladder.
Leisure Counseling	The exploration of what types of leisure/ recreation were of interest to a person before the injury and which are of interest now; how to make the best of leisure time, what recreational resources are available in the community and how to take advantage of them; and what changes have to be made to continue past leisure pursuits.
Leisure Skills	The ability to participate in recreational activities and to independently make effective use of one's leisure time and opportunities.
Lethargic	Awakens with stimulation; drowsy but awake.
Lifelong Living Program	See Program Type
Light Work	Lifting 20 pounds maximum with frequent lifting and/or carrying of objects weighing up to ten pounds, or requiring walking or standing to a significant degree (about six hours a day), or requiring sitting most of the time, but entailing pushing and pulling on arm or leg controls.
Linguistics	The study of human speech, including the units, nature, structure and modification of language.

Locked-In Syndrome	A condition resulting from interruption of motor pathways in the ventral pons, usually by infarction. This disconnection of the motor cells in the spinal cord from controlling signals issued by the brain leaves the patient completely paralyzed and mute, but able to receive and understand sensory stimuli; communication may be possible by code using blinking, or movements of the jaw or eyes, all of which are spared.
Logbook	A diary-like listing of the individual's daily activities which can be used to help remember what happened during the course of the day, names of persons with whom contact occurred, and the order in which events occurred. The brain-injured person, family members and staff are encouraged to make entries. Used to compensate for memory deficits.
Logical Ability	Ability to formulate a general rule or principle which one can use to objectively solve a problem. Also the ability to plan, regulate and control one's own activities.
Lucid Interval	A period shortly after injury when the patient was reported to have talked.
Manpower Development	Cooperative process in which the agencies in the community strive to assure the availability of an adequate present and future supply of qualified personnel to work in programs providing services to handicapped persons.
Medicaid	See appended GLOSSARY OF INSURANCE TERMS.
Medicare	See appended GLOSSARY OF INSURANCE TERMS.
Medically Stable	Reaching a point in medical treatment where life-threatening injuries and disease have been brought under control.
Medium Work	Equivalent to lifting 50 pounds maximum with frequent lifting and/or carrying of objects weighing up to 25 pounds.
Memory	The process of perceiving events, organizing and storing representations of the events and recalling these representations to consciousness at a later time.

Memory, Audio-Visual — Auditory memory is the ability to recall a series of numbers, lists of words, sentences, or paragraphs presented orally. Visual memory requires input of information through visuo-perceptual channels. It refers to the ability to recall text, geometric figures, maps, and photographs. A brain-injured survivor with impaired visual memory may have to refer to a road map numerous times to reach a nearby destination. A brain-injured inpatient may need frequent assistance from staff to locate his room. A patient with impaired auditory memory will likely require frequent reminders of orally-presented task instructions from staff. Notably, information may be encoded in memory using words or visual images independent of the mode of presentation.

Memory, Delayed — The ability to recall information several minutes following presentation. There is no particular specification of the required time interval; typically it is ten minutes or more. This type of memory is most important because patients are often required to recall instructions related to their medical care after hours, days, weeks, or months. For example, patients with impairments in delayed memory may forget where they have left things. Additionally, preserved information in immediate memory becomes part of delayed memory.

Memory, Episodic — Memory for ongoing events in a person's life. More easily impaired than semantic memory, perhaps because rehearsal or repetition tends to be minimal.

Memory, Fund of Information — A type of remote memory as well as an estimate of the amount of information an individual retains about past experiences. The information can include, for example, knowledge regarding current events, politics, and book learning.

Memory, Immediate — The ability to recall numbers, pictures, or words immediately following presentation. Patients with immediate memory problems have difficulty learning new tasks because they cannot remember instructions. Relies upon concentration and attention.

Memory, Learning — Acquisition of new information determined by the extent to which an individual benefits from repetition, rehearsal, or practice. For example, a patient who learns quickly will likely remember an entire set of instructions after hearing them a single time. A patient with severely-impaired learning ability will show little gain in recall after numerous repetitions. Learning and memory are interdependent. If immediate memory is poor, learning will be poor because only a portion of the information will be available for rehearsal/repetition. It is important to note that patients may have intact learning ability, but poor delayed memory. For example, a brain-injured patient may learn a set of instructions after several repetitions, but forget them the next day.

Memory, Long Term — In neuropsychological testing, this refers to recall thirty minutes or longer after presentation. Requires storage and retrieval of information which exceeds the limit of immediate span.

Memory, Recall — Ability to retrieve information without renewed exposure to the stimulus.

Memory, Recognition — Ability to retrieve information when a familiar stimulus is presented.

Memory, Remote — Information an individual correctly recalls from the distant past. There is no specific requirement for the amount of elapsed time, but it is typically more than six months to a year. Preserved information from delayed memory becomes part of remote memory.

Memory, Semantic — Memory for facts, usually learned through repetition.

Memory, Short Term — Primary or 'working' memory, i.e., a limited capacity system that holds up to seven chunks of information over periods of 30 seconds to several minutes.

TIRR BRAIN INJURY GLOSSARY

Mental Competence	The quality or state of being competent; having adequate mental abilities; legally qualified or adequate to manage business affairs. An individual found by a court to be mentally incompetent has a guardian appointed to make business and legal decisions on their behalf.
Mental Disability	All of the recognized forms of mental illness, severe emotional disorders, or mental retardation. Terms such as neurotic, psychotic, and schizophrenic should be reserved for technical medical writing only.
Mental Illness	A condition where there is loss of social and/or vocational skills. Terms such as "mentally deranged", "crazy", "deviant" are not used.
Microcomputer	A small computer: may be used to present information and stimuli to a patient as part of a cognitive rehabilitation program.
Mobility	Ability of an individual to move within, and interact with, the environment, usually involving utilization of public and/or private transportation.
Money Management	Ability to distinguish the different denominations of money, count money, make change, budget.
Monitor, Intensive Care	A TV-like screen with a continuous picture of different wave forms representing different pressures and activities in the body such as blood pressure, intracranial pressure, and EKG. It may also show a corresponding number value for them (digital readout).
Motivation	Requires initiative and refers to the extent to which an individual desires to reach a goal and demonstrates actual follow-through. A greater level of motivation is required for completion of difficult tasks. A brain-injured person with reduced motivation may need frequent cueing to finish dressing even though being able to verbalize the complete procedure.
Motor	Pertaining to movement.

Motor Control	Regulation of the timing and amount of contraction of muscles of the body to produce smooth and coordinated movement. The regulation is carried out by operation of the nervous system.
Motor Control, Fine	Delicate, intricate movements as in writing or playing a piano.
Motor Control, Gross	Large, strong movements as in chopping wood or walking.
Motor Lag	A prolonged delay between stimulus and initiation of motor response.
Motor Planning	Action formulated in the mind before attempting to perform.
Movement Therapy	Using bodily expression, dance and exercise to facilitate movement, self expression and self esteem.
Muscle Tone	Used in clinical practice to describe the resistance of a muscle to being stretched. When the peripheral nerve to a muscle is severed, the muscle becomes flaccid (limp). When nerve fibers in the brain or spinal cord are damaged, the balance between facilitation and inhibition of muscle tone is disturbed. The tone of some muscles may become increased and they resist being stretched - a condition called hypertonicity or spasticity.
Music Therapy	Use of music and singing to develop language and movement skills.
Myelography	A medical test involving injection of dye into the spinal subarachnoid space so that an x-ray of the spinal cord can be taken. Used to detect spinal cord tumors, anatomical defects and disc problems.
NDT	See Neuro Developmental Treatment.
NPO	Latin initials that stand for "Nothing by Mouth". This means no food or liquids for a set period, usually in preparation for certain tests, or when the person cannot safely swallow.
Nasogastric Tube (NG Tube)	A tube which passes through the patient's nose and throat and ends in the patient's

stomach. This tube allows for direct "tube feeding" to maintain the nutritional status of the patient or removal of stomach acids.

Neologism	Nonsense or made-up word used when speaking. The person often does not realize that the word makes no sense.
Neuro Developmental Treatment	A therapeutic approach based on the normal development of movement and emphasizing the restoration of normal movement in performing functional activities.
Neurologist	A physician who specializes in the nervous system and its disorders.
Neurophysiology	The study of the functions of the nervous system.
Neuropsychologist	A psychologist who specializes in evaluating (by tests) brain/behavior relationships, planning training programs to help the patient's brain return to normal functioning and recommending alternative cognitive strategies to minimize the effects of brain injury.
Non-ambulatory	Not able to walk.
Non-disabled	Term for persons without disabilities. The terms normal, able-bodied, healthy, or whole are less appropriate when contrasting those with and those without disabilities.
Non-Purposeful Movement	Movement that a person may make which has no apparent goal.
Normalization	Philosophy that developmentally-disabled individuals should be exposed to patterns and conditions of daily life which are consistent with the norms of society and that training should be provided to enable persons with developmental disabilities to function appropriately in the mainstream of society.
Numerical Ability	Ability to solve numerical problems using the four fundamental rules of arithmetic: addition, subtraction, multiplication, and division.
Nursing Home	A residential facility for the patient who requires supervision in all activities, including assistance with medication, meal

preparation, bathing, dressing, and moving about; the patient may also require special nursing care and/or ongoing therapy. There are nursing homes that provide minimal to maximum care.

Nystagmus — Involuntary horizontal, vertical, or rotary movement of the eyeballs.

Observational Procedure — An organized method of recording what a client does for the purpose of documenting behavior; the emphasis is usually upon productivity, behavior patterns, expressed interest, and worker interaction. Used to gain information concerning a client's overall level of functioning.

O.T. — See Occupational Therapy.

Obtunded — Mental blunting; mild to moderate reduction in alertness.

Occipital Lobe — Region in the back of the brain which processes visual information. Damage to this lobe can cause visual deficits.

Occupational Information — All pertinent facts about a job, or job cluster, which accurately define the characteristics and requirements of the job so that an individual looking for work will have correct, adequate information for making a vocational decision.

Occupational Therapy — Occupational Therapy is the therapeutic use of self-care, work and play activities to increase independent function, enhance development and prevent disability; may include the adaptation of a task or the environment to achieve maximum independence and to enhance the quality of life. The term occupation, as used in occupational therapy, refers to any activity engaged in for evaluating, specifying and treating problems interfering with functional performance.

On-the-Job Training — A planned experience in an actual work situation through which the client, under supervision, learns to perform all job operations of an occupation.

Organization, Cognitive — Using selective attention skills, the patient correctly perceives stimulus attributes or task elements, selects a strategy, monitors use of the strategy and reaches a correct solution.

Low - Level: Those patients who are able to sustain attention and appropriately switch sets. Patients with low level organization ability usually "fall apart" in high-stress situations.

High - Level: Those patients who can deal with multiple pieces of information and integrate them for accomplishing relatively complex tasks. Some patients may still "fall apart" in high-stress situations.

Orientation — An awareness of one's environment and/or situation, and the ability to use this information appropriately in a functional setting.

Orientation, Environment — Knowledge regarding the present environment including where one is at the time of the evaluation. Accurate awareness of place.

Orientation, Left-Right — The ability to discriminate between left and right body parts on oneself and on others, as well as the ability to discriminate between left and right within the environment.

Orientation, Personal — General knowledge related to oneself includes information regarding date of birth, age, name, and location of home.

Orientation, Situational — The ability to accurately describe present circumstances. For example, in the acute stages of injury, brain-injured patients may be unable to respond accurately to questions such as, "Why are you in the hospital?" Situational disorientation is commonly observed during the period of post-traumatic amnesia (PTA).

Orientation, Temporal — Knowledge of the current date, day, month and year. Includes knowledge of facts related to time of day. For example, a disoriented patient asked to name the next meal at 4 PM might say, "breakfast."

Orthopedics — The branch of medicine devoted to the study and treatment of the skeletal system, its joints, muscles and associated structures.

Orthosis	Splint or brace designed to improve function or provide stability.
Orthotist	A skilled craftsman who develops and fits mechanical devices designed to support or supplement a weakened body part, or function, such as a brace, splint or body jacket.
Outcome	The end result.
Outcome, Socio-Ecologic	The Interdisciplinary Special Interest Group (ISIG) Subcommittee on Outcome (of the American Congress of Rehabilitation Medicine) drafted the following statement at its meeting in June 1990: "Brain-injured persons have a capacity to function in the community. Rehabilitation can increase the ability to contribute to society and reduce the negative socio-ecological consequences of brain injury. We are committed to the reliable, valid measures of outcome that consider socio-ecological factors. Outcome measures can be viewed from a variety of perspectives, including impairment, disability and handicap. We recommend that in our Standards of Practice, we not limit measurement of outcome to the realms of impairment or disability. We advocate for outcome measures to include the issue of handicap or the socio-ecological context so that we define outcome around individuals inside of a support system or context."
Outpatient	The patient residing outside the hospital but returning on a regular basis for one or more therapeutic services.
Overnight Drainage Bag (ONDB)	A large thick plastic bag that is connected to a urodrain. It hangs on the bed and is used to collect urine at night or when someone needs to be in bed during the day.
Palliative Care	A program designed to reduce the severity of symptoms and/or decrease their impact on the individual, and to improve the quality of life.
Paraparesis	Weakness of the lower limbs.

TIRR BRAIN INJURY GLOSSARY

Paraphasic Error	Substitution of an incorrect sound (e.g., tree for free) or related word (e.g., chair for bed).
Paraplegia	Paralysis of the legs (from the waist down).
Parapnasias	Use of incorrect words or word combinations.
Parenteral	Not through the alimentary canal (gastrointestinal tract) but rather by injection through some other route, such as subcutaneous, intramuscular or intravenous.
Parietal Lobe	One of the two parietal lobes of the brain located behind the frontal lobe at the top of the brain.
Parietal Lobe, Right	Damage to this area can cause visuo-spatial deficits (e.g., the patient may have difficulty finding their way around new or familiar places).
Parietal Lobe, Left	Damage to this area may disrupt a patient's ability to understand spoken and/or written language.
Pattern of Movement	Motion of particular parts of the body (such as the hand and arm) in a typical, reproducible, sequence and direction.
Perception	The ability to make sense of what one sees, hears, feels, tastes or smells. Perceptual losses are often very subtle, and the patient and/or family may be unaware or them.
Perceptual-Motor	Interaction of the perceptual abilities with motor abilities.
Perseveration	Refers to the inappropriate persistence of a response in a current task which may have been appropriate for a former task. Perseverations may be verbal or motoric.
Persistent Vegetative State (PVS)	A condition in which the patient utters no words and does not follow commands or make any response that is psychologically meaningful. The transition of a person who remains unconscious from a state of 'coma' to one of 'vegetative behaviors' reflects subtle changes over a period of several months from a condition of no response to

the internal or external environment (except reflexively) to a state of wakefulness but with no indication of awareness (cortical function). A patient in this state may have a range of biological responses at the subcortical level such as eye opening (with sleep and wake rhythms) and sometimes the ability to follow with their eyes. Normal levels of blood pressure and respiration (vegetative functions) are maintained automatically. The label 'persistent' is not applicable until the person has been unconscious for a year or more.

Personal Adjustment Training — Process of modifying behavior to conform to measurable criteria based on socially appropriate behavior; process of modifying behavior to enable one to adequately deal with one's environment.

Phlebitis — Inflammation of a vein.

Phonation — The production of sound by means of vocal cord vibration.

Physiatrist — Pronounced Fizz ee at' rist. A physician who specializes in physical medicine and rehabilitation. A physiatrist is an expert in neurologic rehabilitation, trained to diagnose and treat disabling conditions. The physiatrist examines the patient upon admission to assure that medical issues are addressed; provides appropriate medical information to the patient, family members and members of the treatment team. The physiatrist follows the patient closely throughout the admission and oversees the patient's rehabilitation program.

Physical Demands — The physical requirements made on the worker by the specific job/work situation. They include strength (lifting, carrying, pushing, and/or pulling), climbing, or balancing, stooping, kneeling, crouching and/or crawling, reaching, handling, fingering and/or feeling, talking and/or hearing and seeing.

Physical Therapist — The physical therapist evaluates components of movement, including: muscle strength, muscle tone, posture, coordination, endurance, and general mobility. The physical therapist also evaluates the potential for functional movement, such as ability to move in the bed, transfers and walking and then proceeds to establish an individualized treatment program to help the patient achieve functional independence.

Plasticity	The ability of cellular or tissue structures and their resultant function to be influenced by an ongoing activity.
Plateau	A temporary or permanent leveling off in the recovery process.
Policy	See appended GLOSSARY OF INSURANCE TERMS.
Posey Roll	A bar placed on the wheelchair to prevent a person from standing up or falling out.
Posey Vest/ Houdini Jacket	A vest worn to keep the person in bed or in the wheelchair. This is for the person's safety.
Position Sense	The sensory awareness of the location and orientation of body parts without moving them. See kinesthesia and proprioception.
Post Traumatic Amnesia (PTA)	A period of hours, weeks, days or months after the injury when the patient exhibits a loss of day-to-day memory. The patient is unable to store new information and therefore has a decreased ability to learn. Memory of the PTA period is never stored, therefore things that happened during that period cannot be recalled. May also be called Anterograde Amnesia.
Postural Tone, Abnormal	Greater than normal tone of muscles used to hold the body in ordinary positions such as sitting or standing.
Posture	The attitude of the body. Posture is maintained by low-grade, continuous contraction of muscles which counteract the pull of gravity on body parts. Injury to the nervous system can impair the ability to maintain normal posture, for example holding up the head.
Pre-Morbid Condition	Characteristics of an individual present before the disease or injury occurred.

TIRR BRAIN INJURY GLOSSARY

Pre-Screening	The process of reviewing all available pertinent data on referrals to determine the need for additional evaluation.
Prevocational Evaluation	An assessment, prior to work training, of the client's potential as a worker, giving special attention to one's work attitudes and habits, and evidence of personal responsibility.
Primary Care Nurse	The nurse principally responsible for the nursing care of a given patient. The primary care nurse develops and implements a care plan, participates in conferences, collaborates with the patient, the rehabilitation team, and the family, as well as evaluating the outcome of care.
Problem-Solving	Ability of the individual to bring cognitive processes to the consideration of how to accomplish a task.
Problem-Solving Skill	Ability to consider the probable factors that can influence the outcome of each of various solutions to a problem, and to select the most advantageous solution. Patients with deficits in this skill may become "immobilized" when faced with a problem. By being unable to think of possible solutions, they may respond by doing nothing.
Production Work Evaluation	This is a method of evaluating clients through the use of actual industrial work brought into the evaluation facility. It is possible for the evaluation staff to vary all the customary conditions of the real job in an effort to discover difficulties that prevent the client from working effectively.
Prognosis	The prospect as to recovery from a disease or injury as indicated by the nature and symptoms of the case.
Program Manager - Vocational Evaluation (Case Manager)	That professional person who is responsible for the entire evaluation program of an individual client. This includes reviewing all referral information, orientation of the client, scheduling services, planning the individual program, maintaining integration and coordination in the program, maintaining a written case record, holding formal and informal conferences as

appropriate, making the termination decisions, preparing the final report and follow-up.

Program Standards — Requirements that are judged to be necessary for satisfactory operation of a program. At the June, 1990 meeting of the American Congress of Rehabilitation Medicine (ACRM), BRAIN INJURY INTERDISCIPLINARY SPECIAL INTEREST GROUP (ISIG) on STANDARDS proposed that standards could be conceptually organized into the following categories:

- Inpatient Rehabilitation Programs
- Post-acute Treatment Program
  - Residential
  - Day Treatment
- Post-acute Care Program
  - Residential
  - Day Care
- Key Rehabilitation Services
  - Vocational
  - Cognitive
  - Behavioral
  - Academic

Program Type — The following program categories describe the array of organized services available for the rehabilitation of persons with a brain injury:

Acute Rehabilitation — Based in a medical facility; accepts patient as soon as medically stable; focuses on intensive physical and cognitive restorative services in early months after injury; typical length of stay 3-4 months (short term); identifiable team and program with specialized unit.

Behavior Disorders — Patterns of behavior preventing participation in active rehabilitation; destructive patient behavior to self and others; continuum of controlled settings.

Coma Treatment — Accepts patients as soon as active intervention is indicated; Patient functioning at Rancho Los Amigos Scale levels I-IV; and unable to actively participate in therapy;

Day Treatment — Non-residential; intervention across all appropriate disciplines; therapeutic emphasis based in outpatient setting.

TIRR BRAIN INJURY GLOSSARY

Education — Primary, secondary, and higher education programs; realistic academic goals set, based upon professional knowledge of deficits resulting from brain injury.

Employment — Vocational rehabilitation services that are designed to lead to an employment goal; services can range from assessment to basic on-the-job supports; includes one or all of the following: vocational assessment, vocational training, vocational placement, sheltered employment, supported employment.

Homecare — Comprehensive training available for family/caretaker; case management services available prior to home care; team integrated home program.

Independent Living — Community-based to maximize a person's ability to be empowered and self-directed; allows an individual to live in one's own home with maximum personal control over how services are delivered, combined with the opportunity to work as appropriate.

Lifelong Living — For persons discharged from rehabilitation who need ongoing lifetime supports; located in residential or skilled nursing environment; structured activities available on individual and group basis.

Respite/ Recreation — Program allows person and family to adapt psychologically and environmentally to the residual deficits of brain injury; the program is based on a non-interventional model to address socialization, recreation, and respite for the primary care givers needs.

Subacute — May follow a period of acute rehabilitation; not necessarily hospital based; typical length of rehabilitation stay 6-24 months (short to intermediate term); stay based on demonstrated improvement; identifiable team and program with specialized unit.

Transitional Living — Training for living in a setting of greater independence; typical length of stay 4-18 months (short to intermediate term); greater focus on compensation vs. restoration (compensating for skills that cannot be restored); based within the community and has functional emphasis.

Vocational Evaluation — An organized and comprehensive service staffed by specialists who systematically and comprehensively utilize work activities (real or simulated) and/or educational services as the focal point for educational and vocational assessment and exploration. In addition, psychological testing, counseling, social summaries, occupational information, etc., are other evaluation tools that are used. It incorporates the medical, psychological, social, vocational, educational, cultural, and economic data for establishment and attainment of individual goals.

Prone — Lying on one's stomach.

Proprioception — The sensory awareness of the position of body parts with or without movement. Combination of kinesthesia and position sense.

Prosody — The inflections or intonations of speech.

Prosthesis — An artificial substitute for a missing body part, such as an arm or leg, eye or tooth, used for functional or cosmetic reasons or both.

Prosthetist — A skilled craftsman who designs and makes artificial replacements for missing body parts, for example, an artificial leg.

Proximal — Next to, or nearest, the point of attachment.

Proximal Instability — Weakness of muscles of the trunk, shoulder girdle or hip girdle which causes poor posture, abnormal movement of the arms or legs and the inability to hold one's head up. Strength of muscles of the hands or legs may be normal.

Psychologist — A professional specializing in counselling, including adjustment to disability. Psychologists use tests to identify personality and cognitive functioning. This information is shared with team members to assure consistency in approaches. The psychologist may provide individual or group psychotherapy for the purpose of cognitive retraining, management

	of behavior and the development of coping skills by the patient and members of the family.
Psychometric Instruments	Standardized tests (utilizing paper and pencil) which measure mental functioning.
Psychomotor Skills	Skills that involve both mental and muscular ability such as playing sports or other activities where practice or concentration is involved.
Psychosocial Skills	Refers to the individual's adjustment to the injury (and resulting disability) and one's ability to relate to others. Includes feelings about self, sexuality and the resulting behaviors.
Ptosis	Drooping of a body part, such as the upper eyelid, from paralysis, or drooping of visceral organs from weakness of the abdominal muscles.
Purposeful Movement	Motor activity with an apparent goal.
P.A.	Physician's Assistant.
P.T.	See Physical Therapist
PTA	See post-traumatic amnesia.
Quadriparesis	Weakness of all four limbs.
Quadriplegia	Paralysis of all four limbs (from the neck down). British authors often use the prefix "tetra" to mean four, so they may describe a patient as having tetraplegia.
Quality of Life	A rating of what kind of existence a person experiences. In estimating the quality of life the following items are usually considered: 1) activities of daily life; 2) mobility and organization of living arrangements; 3) social relationships; 4) work or leisure activities; 5) present satisfaction; and 6) future prospects.
R.T.	See Respiratory Therapist.
Random Movement	An action or process of moving without obvious aim, purpose, or reason.
Range of Motion (ROM)	Refers to movement of a joint (important to prevent contractures).

Range of Motion, Active	The muscles around the joint do the work to move it.
Range of Motion, Passive	Movement of a joint by means other than contraction of the muscles around that joint; e.g., someone else moves the joint.
Reasoning, Abstract	Requires that the individual recognize a phrase that has multiple meanings and select the meaning most appropriate to a given situation. The term "abstract" typically refers to concepts not readily apparent from the physical attributes of an object or situation.
Reasoning, Association	A skill dependent on a patient's ability to determine the relationship between objects and concepts. A patient with impairment may touch a hot stove, failing to realize that pain is associated with touching a heated burner. Similarly, a patient given a knife, spoon, fork, and baseball may not be able to discriminate which of the objects "does not belong."
Reasoning, Categorization	The ability to sort or group objects and concepts based on the shared attribute(s) and apply a label depicting the attribute(s). Task difficulty is greater in circumstances requiring formulation of new categories. Impaired patients may have difficulty sorting clothes or choosing items for a balanced meal. Categorization is similar to association in that patients must understand the relationship between objects or concepts. However, categorization requires an extra step; the ability to provide a label describing the group of objects or concepts.
Reasoning, Cause and Effect	The ability to perceive and anticipate the consequences of a given action or statement. For example, a patient may sit for a long period in a darkened room without realizing that flipping a light switch will cause the light to turn on. A patient may turn the oven up to make a cake cook faster, not realizing that the increased heat will simply cause the food to burn.
Reasoning, Concrete	Involves the ability to understand the literal meaning of a phrase.

TIRR BRAIN INJURY GLOSSARY

Reasoning, Generalization — The ability to take information, rules and strategies learned about one situation and apply them appropriately to other, similar situations. For example, a patient who learns to lock his wheelchair brakes in physical therapy may not lock the brakes while sitting in his room.

Reasoning, Organization — The ability to arrange or group information in a manner which improves task efficiency. Patients who lack organizational skills often demonstrate a sense of purposelessness and have difficulty effectively utilizing non-structured time. They have difficulty completing a puzzle or arranging materials to cook or shower.

Reasoning, Problem-Solving — The ability to analyze information related to a given situation and generate appropriate response options. Problem-solving is a sequential process that typically proceeds as follows: identification of problem; generation of response options; evaluation of response option appropriateness; selection and testing of first option; analysis as to whether solution has been reached. A patient may discontinue making a cup of coffee because the sugar bowl is empty, even though sugar is readily available in a nearby cabinet. A patient may easily navigate his way into a room crowded with furniture, but request staff assistance to navigate his way out.

Reasoning, Sequencing — The ability to organize information or objects according to specified rules, or the ability to arrange information or objects in a logical, progressive manner. Nearly every activity, including work and leisure tasks, requires sequencing. For example, in cooking certain foods it is important that ingredients be added and mixed in a specified order; in dressing, undergarments must be put on prior to outergarments.

Recreation Supervisor — Individual within the facility responsible for developing a program to assist handicapped individuals to plan and manage their leisure activities; may

	also schedule specific activities and coordinate program with existing community resources.
Referral	The process of directing a client to an agency for services.
Referral Data	Data about the client obtained from other specialists, persons, and agencies that is obtained verbally or through such documents as psychometrics, terminal reports, medical reports, intake, and social service reports.
Referral Source	That person or facility who refers a client for services. This includes, but is not limited to, service agencies such as vocational rehabilitation, physicians, industry, insurance companies, employment agencies, community action groups, and potential clients themselves.
Referring Agency	The agency which sends or directs the client for services.
Refrig Bag	Device used to help keep males dry when they are incontinent. It is a small plastic bag filled with absorbent tissue that is secured around the penis.
Rehabilitation	Comprehensive program to reduce/overcome deficits following injury or illness, and to assist the individual to attain the optimal level of mental and physical ability.
Rehabilitation Counselor	Also called Vocational Counselor. A specialist in social and vocational issues who helps the patient develop the skills and aptitudes necessary for return to work and the community.
Rehabilitation Engineering	Use of technical advances, physics, computer science and other scientific devices to aid in improving the quality of life for the handicapped person, e.g., computerized communication boards, mechanically-assisted wheelchairs.
Rehabilitation Facility	Agency of multiple, coordinated services designed to minimize for the individual the handicapping effects one's his physical,

	mental, social, and/or vocational impairment, and to help realize individual potential.
Rehabilitation Nurse	A nurse specializing in rehabilitation techniques as well as basic nursing care. Nurses assist the patient and family in acquiring new information, developing skills, achieving competence and exhibiting behaviors that contribute to the attainment of a healthy state.
Rehabilitation Objective	A goal of the comprehensive restoration of an individual to the best possible level of functioning following a physical, mental, or emotional disorder.
Rehabilitation Process	A planned, orderly sequence of services related to the total needs of the handicapped individual and designed to assist one to realize maximum potential for useful and productive activity.
Rehabilitation Team	An organized group of health care specialists, who focus on providing a logical, practical and complete rehabilitation plan for the patient. Upon admission to the rehabilitation hospital, the patient is evaluated by each team member who defines both short-term and long-term goals for the patient's rehabilitation. Meetings of the rehabilitation team (sometimes called "rounds") are held regularly to discuss the patient's progress and, if necessary, to redefine the goals. Additional family conferences may also be scheduled.
Remediation	The process of decreasing a handicap by challenging the individual to improve deficient skills.
Report-Vocational Evaluation	A well planned, carefully written means of communicating vital vocational information about a client. It is a studied, permanent record of significant vocational data observed as a client and an evaluator interact in various types of work or work-like situations. It puts the plan, action, findings, logic, and interpretation of the evaluation in writing. It usually includes a description of the client's work traits and how they compare to minimal requirements of selected jobs or work

areas, physical capacities, learning ability, personal characteristics, social competence, other vocational factors, and recommendation for further services. It may also provide a prescriptive-descriptive sequence of experiences which are aimed at maximizing an individual's vocational potential.

Respirator/Ventilator — A machine that does the breathing work for the unresponsive patient. It serves to deliver air in the appropriate percentage of oxygen and at the appropriate rate. The air is also humidified by the respirator.

Respite Care — A means for taking over the care of a patient temporarily (a few hours up to a few days) to provide a period of relief for the primary caregiver.

Response Control — Development of the ability to recognize and suppress abnormal behaviors in one's self. Two behaviors fall within this category: impulse control, and perseveration.

Respiratory Therapist — The respiratory therapist is concerned with helping the patient breathe adequately by use of various machines as well as techniques to keep the airway clear of secretions.

Retrograde Amnesia — Inability to recall events prior to the accident; may be a specific span of time or type of information.

S.T. — See Speech and Hearing Therapist.

Scanning — The active search of the environment for information; usually refers to "visual scanning" which is a skill used in reading, driving and many daily activities.

Scotoma — Area of blindness of varying size anywhere within the visual fields.

Secondary Insults — Secondary or delayed brain injury; includes all events other than the mechanical injury sustained at the time of impact. Secondary phenomena may be divided into systemic and intracranial insults. Systemic insults include hypoxemia, anemia, hypotension, hypercarbia, hyperthermia, and electrolyte imbalance.

Sedentary Work — Equivalent to lifting ten pounds maximum with occasional lifting and/or carrying small objects. While mostly done sitting, a certain amount of walking and standing is often necessary in carrying out job duties.

Seizure — An uncontrolled discharge of nerve cells which may spread to other cells nearby or throughout the entire brain. It usually lasts only a few minutes. It may be associated with loss of consciousness, loss of bowel and bladder control and tremors. May also cause aggressive or other behavioral change.

Selective Attention — Ability to focus on the most important aspect of a situation without becoming distracted.

Selective Placement — Placement where a client can work in a situation where provisions are made by the employer to meet the client's special needs.

Sensation — Feeling stimuli which activate sensory organs of the body, such as touch, temperature, pressure and pain. Also seeing, hearing, smelling and tasting.

Sensorimotor — Refers to all aspects of movement and sensation and the interaction of the two.

Sensory Deprivation — A situation or environment where usual sensory stimuli, such as noise and light, as well as human contact, are absent or substantially decreased. In the case of noise, it may be masked by a continuous dull noise.

Sensory Integration — Interaction of two or more sensory processes in a manner which enhances the adaptiveness of the brain.

Sensory Stimulation — Arousing the brain through any of the senses.

Sequencing — Reading, listening, expressing thoughts, describing events or contracting muscles in an orderly and meaningful manner.

Sexuality Counseling — Using supportive techniques and special methods to help brain-injured survivors and their families deal with special and intimate relationship issues.

Sheltered Workshop — A work setting certified as such by the Wage & Hour Division. It provides transitional and/or long-term employment in a controlled and protected working environment for those who are unable either to compete or to function in the open job market due to their handicap. May provide vocational evaluation and work adjustment services.

Shock, Circulatory — A clinical condition characterized by signs and symptoms which arise when the cardiac output is insufficient to fill the arterial tree with blood under sufficient pressure to provide organs and tissues with adequate blood flow.

Shunt — A procedure to draw off excessive fluid in the brain. A surgically-placed tube running from the ventricles which deposits fluid into either the abdominal cavity, heart or large veins of the neck.

Simulated Job Station — A work setting which has the following characteristics: 1) replication of all aspects of a job (not limited to job tasks) or a work process as realistically as possible; 2) does not necessarily require payment to the client; 3) the setting is controlled by the evaluator; and 4) it is located within the evaluation facility.

Single Trait Work Samples — Assesses a single worker trait or characteristic. It may have relevance to a specific job or many jobs, but it is intended to assess a single, isolated factor.

Skill Training — Teaching an individual how to perform the operations of a particular occupation; distinguished from personal adjustment training, work adjustment, and the acquisition of basic employability.

Skill Remediation — A process in which the aim is to improve skills that have been imperfectly or inadequately learned.

Skull Fracture — The breaking of the bones surrounding the brain. A depressed skull fracture is one in which the broken bone exerts pressure on the brain.

Small Stature
Used to refer to very small persons; more socially acceptable than the terms dwarf or midget. Dwarfism is an accepted medical term, but it should not be used in general conversation.

Social Adjustment Group
A structured group experience that offers individuals opportunities for the redirection of energies toward positive social goals, raising of levels of aspiration, and/or reduction of maladaptive behavior patterns.

Social Adjustment Training
Structured program designed to assist the handicapped individual to interact with individuals and groups within the community in an acceptable manner.

Social Assessment
A social assessment includes general background data, description of family or other support group resources -- including emotional, financial and environment resources, their availability to the patient, and the patient's position and role in the family (child, parent, spouse) -- and educational and employment history. Also included are such topics as interests, life-style, friendships, goals, ambitions, personality traits, positive and/or negative relationships and previous problems (such as medical, psychiatric, drug abuse, alcohol). The assessment attempts to reveal the patient's and the family's level of understanding of the patient's current condition, probable long-range outcome, expectations of rehabilitation, degree of disruption in family functioning that the disability has produced, and the ability and interest of the patient and family members to adjust to changed circumstances.

Social Worker
The social worker serves as a liaison between the professional team and other parties concerned with the patient, including: the family, funding sources, friends and representatives of past or future placements. An important role of the social worker is to help ensure that if home placement does not materialize, or if home placement is not indicated, the social worker provides assistance to the patient and family for finding other alternatives.

TIRR BRAIN INJURY GLOSSARY

"Space Boots" (Spenco Boots)	Padded support devices made of lamb's wool used to position the feet and ankles of the patient. Without this support and alignment, patients who are unconscious for long periods may develop deformities limiting future movement.
Spasticity	An involuntary increase in muscle tone (tension) that occurs following injury to the brain or spinal cord, causing the muscles to resist being moved. Characteristics may include increase in deep tendon reflexes, resistance to passive stretch, clasp knife phenomenon, and clonus.
Spatial Ability	Ability to perceive the construction of an object in both two and three dimensions. Spatial ability is composed of four components: the ability to perceive a static figure in different positions, the ability to interpret and duplicate the movements between various parts of a figure, the ability to perceive the relationship between an object and a person's own body sphere, and the ability to interpret the person's body as an object in space.
Special	Describes that which is different or uncommon about any person. This term should not be used to describe persons with disabilities (except when citing laws or regulations).
Specialty Services	Categories identified by the National Head Injury Foundation (NHIF) to classify frequently requested services. These services include: respirator-dependent, substance abuse, driver education, evaluation, visually-impaired and Spanish translation.
Specific Learning Disability	Permanent condition that affects the way individuals with average or above-average intelligence take in, retain, and express information. The term "specific" is preferred, because it emphasizes that only certain learning processes are affected.
Speech Disorder	A condition where a person has limited or difficult speech patterns.

Speech and Hearing Therapist — The speech pathologist and audiologist identifies problem areas of visual (seeing) and auditory (hearing) comprehension, attention, memory (recent and past), language skills, writing skills and reading skills. The information gathered by the speech and hearing specialist is valuable to other team members; for example, whether or not to use reading as a means of communicating information to the patient. The speech therapist provides instruction and practice in improving skills in comprehension and communication.

Speech-Language Pathology Services — A continuum of services including prevention, identification, diagnosis, consultation, and treatment of patients regarding speech, language, oral and pharyngeal sensorimotor function.

Spontaneous Movement — A reaction resulting from a natural impulse without obvious planning or premeditation.

Spontaneous Recovery — The recovery which occurs as damage to body tissues heals. This type of recovery occurs with or without rehabilitation and it is very difficult to know how much improvement is spontaneous and how much is due to rehabilitative interventions. However, when the recovery is guided by an experienced rehabilitation team, complications can be anticipated and minimized; the return of function can be channeled in useful directions and in progressive steps so that the eventual outcome is the best that is possible.

Staff Conferences (Staffing) — Formal or informal conferences held by the staff working with client to review progress of the individual, develop further plans, maintain integration and coordination of the client's programs, and to make recommendations as to further action needed by and for the client.

Standards — A set of criteria used to measure the merit of an agency's program.

Status Epilepticus — Continuous seizures; may produce permanent brain damage.

Stimulus — That which causes sensation (i.e., light for vision, salt for taste, sound for hearing, etc.). When a patient begins to emerge from coma, an organized program of controlled stimulation is sometimes used to begin "exercising" the brain. However, when a patient becomes agitated, the amount and intensity of stimulation should be limited (e.g., only one task for one sense at a time).

Strabismus, External (III)	Outward turning of the eye which may be due to a lesion of the oculomotor nerve causing paralysis of the medial rectus muscle.
Strabismus, Internal	Inward turning of the eye which may be due to a lesion of the abducens nerve (VI) causing paralysis of the lateral rectus muscle.
Stupor	Deep sleep; unresponsive but can be awakened with repeated, noxious stimulation. Awareness is depressed but present.
Subacute	The prefix "sub" means under, below, near or less than complete; "acute" means sharp, severe; having a sudden onset, sharp rise and short course. Thus, a subacute condition is one which has not reached or has already passed through the acute phase.
Subacute Program	See Program Type
Subarachnoid Screw	Also Subarachnoid Bolt. A device for measuring intracranial pressure which is screwed through a hole in the skull and rests on the surface of the brain.
Subdural	Beneath the dura (tough membrane) covering the brain and spinal cord.
Substance Abuse Program	A service offered by an agency to deal with chemical dependency of an individual. The dependency may have occurred prior to the brain injury or subsequent to the brain injury.
Supervision	Refers to the assistance provided when an individual requires no physical help but requires another person nearby for safety.
Close	Assistant stands close to person, ready to give assistance if needed.

Distant	Assistant can see the person and offer verbal assistance but is not close enough to touch the person.
Supine	Lying on one's back.
Support Group	A group established for families and/or persons with disabilities to discuss the problems they may be having in coping with their life situation and to seek solutions to these problems.
Support Hose	Anti-embolic stockings. Tight knee or thigh-high stockings that support the leg muscles and thus help prevent pooling of blood in veins of the legs.
Supported Employment	Competitive work in integrated work settings for individuals with severe handicaps for whom competitive employment has not traditionally occurred, or for whom competitive employment has been interrupted as a result of severe disability, and who, because of the handicaps, need ongoing support services to perform that work.
Suppository	Medicine contained in a capsule which is inserted into the rectum so that the Medicine can be absorbed into the blood stream.
Swan-Ganz Catheter	A catheter (tube) similar to the central venous pressure (CVP) line. It is used to measure blood pressure and blood gas concentrations in the right side of the heart, in vessels of the lungs and in the left side of the heart.
Synergy (movement)	Combined action of two or more muscles to form a pattern of movement.
Synthesizing	The process by which information from all resources is combined into a meaningful whole to determine approaches and directions.
Tactile Defensiveness	Being overly sensitive to touch; withdrawing, crying, yelling or striking when one is touched.
Tactile Discrimination	The ability to differentiate information received through the sense of touch. Sharp/dull discrimination - ability to distinguish between sharp and dull stimuli;

	Two-point discrimination - the ability to recognize two points applied to the skin simultaneously as distinct from one single point.
Task Analysis	Breakdown of a particular job into its component parts; information gained from task analysis can be utilized to develop training curricula or to price a product or service.
TEDS	See Support Hose
Telegraphic Speech	Speech which sounds like a telegram. Only the main words of a sentence (nouns, verbs) are present; the small words (ifs, ands, buts,) are missing. This type of speech often gets the message across.
Temperament	Personal traits consisting of the individual's characteristic mode or inclination of emotional response.
Temporal Lobes	There are two temporal lobes, one on each side of the brain located at about the level of the ears. These lobes allow a person to tell one smell from another and one sound from another. They also help in sorting new information and are believed to be responsible for short-term memory.
Right Lobe	Mainly involved in visual memory (i.e., memory for pictures and faces).
Left Lobe	Mainly involved in verbal memory (i.e., memory for words and names).
Third Party Funding	Reimbursement for services rendered to a person in which an entity other than the recipient of the services is responsible for the payments, i.e., an insurance company.
Thrombus	Blood clot
Time Study	Detailed, scientific analysis of time taken by a worker to perform each segment of a specific task/job, and the hand and body movements made in performing the task/job. Such a study may be made for the purpose of determing the most efficient method for doing the task/job, or to evaluate the task/job to establish a work standard or to set a wage.

Timed Voiding	Bladder training program where the person goes to the toilet at regular intervals whether feeling the urge to urinate or not. The goal is bladder contingency through better control and timing.
Tone, Muscle	The tension in resting muscles and the amount of resistance that is felt when a muscle is moved.
Tracheostomy	A temporary surgical opening at the front of the throat providing access to the trachea or windpipe to assist in breathing.
Tracking, Visual	Visually following an object as it moves through space.
Traction	A weighted traction setup composed of pulleys and lines used in the care of the patient with broken legs or spine. After the repair of the fractures and application of the appropriate casts, weights are used to keep the bones correctly aligned.
Training Environment	Refers to the setting in which the emphasis is on the learning and acquisition of skills or competencies.
Transducer	A sensitive electronic device which detects bodily functions, such as heart rate and blood pressure, and transmits signals representing those functions to a monitor so that they can be observed.
Transfer	Moving one's body between wheelchair and bed, toilet, mat, or car with or without the assistance of another person.
Transitional Living Program	See Program Type.
Treatment Modalities	Various therapy techniques.
Treatment Protocol	The written treatment plan specifying the procedures to be followed by the treatment team.
Tremor, Intention	Course, rhythmical movements of a body part that become intensified the harder one tries to control them.

Tremor, Resting — Rhythmical movements present at rest and may be diminished during voluntary movement.

Unconditional Positive Regard — Absolute or unreserved acceptance and respect.

Unilateral — Pertaining to only one side.

Unilateral Neglect — Paying little or no attention to things on one side of the body. This usually occurs on the side opposite from the location of the injury to the brain because nerve fibers from the brain typically cross before innervating body structures. In extreme cases, the patient may not bathe, dress or acknowledge one side of the body.

Urinary Tract Infection — When bacteria have reproduced to a large number in the bladder. This can cause fever, chills, burning on urination, urgency, frequency, incontinence, or foul smelling urine.

Urodrain — A type of external urine-collecting device for men.

Vegetative State — Return of wakefulness but not accompanied by cognitive function; eyes open to verbal stimuli; does not localize motor responses; autonomic functions preserved. Sleep-wake cycles exist. See Persistent Vegetative State.

Ventricles, Brain — Four natural cavities in the brain which are filled with cerebrospinal fluid. The outline of one or more of these cavities may change when a space-occupying lesion (hemorrhage, tumor) has developed in a lobe of the brain.

Ventriculostomy — A procedure for measuring intracranial pressure by placing a measuring device within one of the fluid-filled, hollow chambers of the brain.

Verbal Ability — Composed of verbal understanding and verbal fluency. Verbal understanding is the ability of an individual to understand the subtleties and meaning of words; verbal fluency is the ability to imagine, process and say words without associating them with any particular object. Also the ability to communicate by talking, writing, listening and reading.

Verbal Apraxia — Impaired control of proper sequencing of muscles used in speech (tongue, lips, jaw muscles, vocal cords). These muscles are not weak but their control is defective. Speech is labored and characterized by sound reversals, additions and word approximations.

Verbal Fluency — The ability to produce words.

Verbal Request — Asking a person for a specified response.

Vestibular — Pertaining to the vestibular system in the middle ear and the brain which senses movements of the head. Disorders of the vestibular system can lead to dizziness, poor regulation of postural muscle tone and inability to detect quick movements of the head.

Visual Field Defect — Inability to see objects located in a specific region of the field of view ordinarily received by each eye. Often the blind region includes everything in the right half or left half of the visual field.

Visual Imagery — The use of mental pictures to aid in recall.

Visual Perception — The ability to recognize and discriminate between visual stimuli and to interpret these stimuli through association with earlier experiences. For example, to separate a figure from a background, to synthesize the contents of a picture and to interpret the invariability of an object which is seen from different directions.

Visually-Impaired — Generic term preferred by some individuals to refer to all degrees of vision loss.

Visually-Impaired Program — A service offered by a program to deal with an individual who is blind. The blindness may have occurred prior to a brain injury or as a result of a brain injury.

Vocation — A summons or strong inclination to a particular state or course of action grounded in interest, ability, need, and opportunities; the work in which a person is regularly employed.

Vocational Adjustment Center	A rehabilitation facility that is to facilitate the transition to employment of vocationally-handicapped persons who experience emotional, mental, physical, or social disability. Its vocational treatment goals may either be an improvement in the capacity to function productively, or in the ability to secure appropriate employment, or in the capacity to adapt on the job. These changes may be accomplished by increasing psychological work capacity, by modifying a client's vocational pattern to conform to the stereotype of a good worker (the work personality), or by developing personality characteristics which are needed to adjust to the requirements of the job.
Vocational Counseling	Process of assisting a person to understand vocational liabilities and assets, provide occupational information to assist one in choosing an occupation suitable to one's interests and liabilities.
Vocational Counselor	Individual who does vocational counseling (Also, see Rehabilitation Counselor).
Vocational Education	Courses of study, under supervision and control, which lead to proficiency in specific trades or business occupations.
Vocational Evaluation	A comprehensive process that systematically utilizes work, real or simulated, as the focal point for assessment and vocational exploration, the purpose of which is to assist individuals in vocational development. Vocational evaluation incorporates medical, psychological, social, vocational, educational, cultural, and economic data in the attainment of the goals of the evaluation process.
Vocational Evaluation Department	A program organized to provide vocational evaluation services as established by standards.
Vocational Evaluation Program Manager (Case Manager)	The professional responsible for the entire evaluation program of an individual client. This includes reviewing all referral information,

orientation of the client, scheduling services, planning the individual program, maintaining integration and coordination in his program, maintaining a written case record, holding formal and informal conferences as appropriate, making the termination decision, preparing the final report and follow-up.

Vocational Evaluation Services	Those services provided to accomplish vocational evaluation according to established standards.
Vocational Evaluation Unit (Department)	Is the staff, plant, and equipment necessary to carry out a vocational evaluation program.
Vocational Evaluator	The individual staff member responsible for carrying out a vocational evaluation.
Vocational Objective	A specific, job-related, time-oriented statement which is set forth at the beginning of, and may be modified during, the client's rehabilitation program.
Vocational Rehabilitation Process	Providing, in a coordinated manner, those services deemed appropriate to the needs of a handicapped individual, and designed to achieve objectives directed toward the realization of the individual's maximum physical, social, mental, and vocational potential.
Vocational Training	The learning and acquisition of skills or competencies whose ultimate objective is the preparation of students for employment.
Voluntary or Volitional Movement	Refers to movement purposefully made by the person.
Volunteer	Individual who freely contributes time and talents to an agency engaged in providing services to people, without remuneration commensurate with the value of services rendered by the volunteer.
Wagner-O'Day	Common name for Public Law 92-28 which directs the purchase by the Federal Government of selected commodities and services from qualified workshops serving blind and other severely handicapped individuals, with the objective of

	increasing the employment opportunities for these individuals.
Word Retrieval Deficit	Difficulty recalling a specific word or words.
Work Activity Center	A workshop, or physically-separate department of a workshop, having a planned, identifiable program designed exclusively to provide therapeutic activity for handicapped workers whose physical or mental impairment is so severe as to make their production inconsequential.
Work Adjustment	An individualized, structured and planned, closely supervised, remedial work experience designed to promote the acquisition of good work habits, to increase physical and emotional tolerance for work activity and interpersonal relationships, and to modify aptitudes and behaviors which inhibit the satisfactory performance of work.
Work Aptitude	One's natural ability or general suitability to work; sometimes refers to a measure of that ability.
Worker's Compensation	See appended GLOSSARY OF INSURANCE TERMS.
Work Environment Work Setting	Surroundings in and the conditions under which an individual performs occupational duties including lighting, equipment, cleanliness, and type of supervision.
Work Families	See Job Clusters.
Work Habits	Those aspects of behavior in a work setting that enable a person to meet the demands of a job in accordance to employment standards. This includes such areas as: attendance, punctuality, hygiene, social behavior, team work, cooperation, ability to accept constructive criticism, ability to accept supervision, effort, initiative, perseverance, dependability, meeting work schedules, attention to detail, housekeeping, neatness in work performed, careful with materials and property, and safety awareness.

Work Personality	The individual's traits, habits, and attitudes related to the concept of employment, and one's reaction to that concept.
Work Station	Physical site where a production operation is performed (Syn: Job Station).
Work Tolerance	Ability to sustain a work effort for a prolonged period of time; ability to maintain a steady flow of production at an acceptable pace and acceptable level of quality; ability to handle a certain amount of pressure.
Worker Functions	The functioning of the worker in relationship to a specific set of tasks. A combination of the highest function which the worker performs in relation to data, people, and things, expresses the total level of complexity of the job/worker situation.
Worker Trait	The requirements made of the worker in terms of aptitudes, general educational development, vocational preparation, physical demands, and personal traits. These are reflected in: training time, aptitudes, temperaments, interests, physical demands, and environmental conditions.
Workmen's Compensation	Insurance programs, under state auspices or control, except for Federal employees and certain maritime workers, to provide financial resources for medical care and lost wages and earning power resulting from industrial accidents, and from illnesses resulting from employment.
Work Sample	A well defined work activity involving tasks, materials, and tools which are identical or similar to those in an actual job or cluster of jobs. It is used to assess an individual's vocational aptitude, worker characteristics, and vocational interest. See also: Job Task.
Work Sample Normed In Industrial Setting	A work sample for which the available norms include the empirical norm reference of a population employed in a competitive industrial setting.

TIRR BRAIN INJURY GLOSSARY

GLOSSARY OF INSURANCE TERMS

Accident	An event causing loss, which takes place without being expected. In most cases the accident can be characterized with regard to time and place of occurrence.
Adjuster	A person who handles claims. This term is becoming obsolete because it's connotation is often negative and misunderstood (see Claims Service Representative).
Administrative Services Only Plan	An arrangement under which an insurance carrier or an independent organization will, for a fee, handle the administration of claims, benefits, and other administrative functions of a self-insured group.
Aggregate Indemnity	The maximum dollar amount that may be collected for any disability, or period of disability, under the policy.
Benefits	The amount payable by the insurance company to a claimant, assignee, or beneficiary under each coverage.
Blanket Medical Expense	A provision which entitles the insured person to collect up to a maximum established in the policy for all hospital and medical expenses incurred, without any limitation on individual types of medical expenses.
Carrier	The insurance company or the one who agrees to pay the losses. The carrier may be organized as a company (either stock, mutual, or reciprocal), or as an Association of Underwriters.
Case Reserve	The dollar amount stated in a claim file which represents the estimate of the amount unpaid.
Claim	A request for payment of reparation for a loss covered by an insurance contract.
Claimant	One who seeks a claim.
Claims Service Representative	A person who investigates losses and settles claims for an insurance carrier or the insured. A term preferred to adjuster.

TIRR BRAIN INJURY GLOSSARY

Coinsurance	A policy provision frequently found in major medical insurance, by which both the insured person and the insurer share the covered losses under a policy in a specified ratio.
Comprehensive Major Medical Insurance	A policy designed to give the protection offered by both a basic and a major medical health insurance policy. It is characterized by a low deductible amount, a coinsurance feature, and high maximum benefits.
Contributory	A group insurance plan issued to an employer under which both the employer and employee contribute to the cost of the plan; 75% of the eligible employees must be insured.
Deductible	The amount of covered charges incurred by the protected person which must be assumed or paid by the insured before benefits by the insurance carrier become payable.
Disability	The state of being disabled from earning full wages at the work at which the employee was last employed.
Disability Income Insurance	A form of health insurance that provides periodic payments to replace income when an insured person is unable to work as a result of illness, injury, or disease.
Dismemberment	Loss of a body member(s), or use thereof, or loss of sight due to injury.
Double Indemnity	A policy provision usually associated with death, which doubles payment of a designated benefit when certain kinds of accidents occur.
Duplication of Benefits	Overlapping or identical coverage of the same insured under two or more health plans, usually the result of contracts of different insurance companies, service organizations, or prepayment plans; also know as multiple coverage.
Elimination Period	A period of time between the period of disability and the start of disability income insurance benefits, during which no benefits are payable (see Waiting Period).

TIRR BRAIN INJURY GLOSSARY

Evidence of Insurability	Any statement of proof of a person's physical condition and/or other factual information affecting his/her acceptance for insurance.
Exclusions	Specific conditions or circumstances listed in the policy for which the policy will not provide benefit payments.
Health Insurance	Protection which provides payment of benefits for covered sickness or injury. Included under this heading are various types of insurance such as accident insurance, disability income insurance, medical expense insurance, and accidental death and dismemberment insurance.
Impairment	The inability or lessened ability to function in the performance of work duties because of injury or illness from a work-related accident or disease.
Injury	Harm to a worker subject to treatment and/or compensable under workers' compensation.
Insured	The person, organization or other entity who purchases insurance.
Insurer	The insurance company or any other organization which assumes the risk and provides the policy to the insured.
Lapse	Termination of a policy upon the policyholder's failure to pay the premium within the time required.
Medicaid	State programs of public assistance to persons regardless of age whose income and resources are insufficient to pay for health care. Provided under Title XIX of the Federal Social Security Act of 1966.
Medicare	The hospital insurance system and the supplementary medical insurance for disabled or aged persons created by the 1965 amendments to the Social Security Act.
Morbidity	The incidence and severity of sicknesses and accidents in a well-defined class or classes of people.

TIRR BRAIN INJURY GLOSSARY

Nondisabling Injury	An injury which may require medical care, but does not result in loss of working time or income.
Occupational Disease	Any disease or specified diseases that are common to or a result of a particular occupation or specific work environment.
Occupational Hazard	Occupations that expose the insured to greater than normal physical dangers by the very nature of the work in which the insured is engaged, and the varying periods of absence from the occupation, due to the disability, that can be expected.
Occurrence	Any incident or happening involving possible loss to a policyholder.
Partial Disability	The result of an illness or injury which prevents an insured from performing one or more of the functions of his/her regular job.
Policy	The legal document issued by the company to the policyholder which outlines the conditions and terms of the insurance.
Policyholder	One who owns an insurance policy.
Pre-Existing Condition	A physical and/or mental condition of an insured which first manifested itself prior to the issuance of the individual policy or which existed prior to issuance and for which treatment was received.
Premium	The periodic payment required to keep a policy in force.
Rehabilitation	Restoration of a totally-disabled person to a meaningful occupation. A provision in some long-term disability policies that provides for continuation of benefits or other financial assistance while a totally-disabled insured is retraining or attempting to resume productive employment.
Residual Disability Benefit	A provision in an insurance policy that provides benefits in proportion to a reduction of earnings as a result of disability, as opposed to the inability to work full-time.
Rider	A document which amends the policy or certificate. It may increase or decrease

	benefits, waive the conditions of coverage, or in any other way amend the original contract.
Risk	The uncertainty of loss with respect to person, liability, or the property of the insured.
Self-Administration	The procedure where an employer maintains all records regarding the employees covered under a group insurance plan.
Self-Insurer	An employer who can meet the state legal and financial requirements to assume all risks and pay for the losses, although the employer may contract with an insurance carrier or others to provide certain essential services.
Third-Party Administration	Administration of a group insurance plan by some person or firm other than the insurer or the policyholder.
Tort Liability	The legal requirement that a person responsible, or at fault, shall pay for the damages and injuries caused.
Total Disability	An illness or injury that prevents an insured person from continuously performing every duty pertaining to his/her occupation or engaging in any other type of work.
Underwriter	The term generally is used for either: a) a company that receives the premiums and accepts responsibility for the fulfillment of the insurance policy contract; b) the company employee who decides whether or not the insurance company should assume a particular risk; or c) the agent who sells the policy.
Uninsurable Risk	One not acceptable for insurance due to excessive risk.
Waiting Period	The length of time an employee must wait from date of employment or application for coverage, to the date that the insurance policy is effective.
Waiver	An agreement attached to a policy that exempts from coverage certain disabilities or injuries which are normally covered by the policy.

Workers' Compensation	The social insurance system for industrial and work injury regulated primarily among separate states, but regulated in certain specified occupations by the federal government.
Workers' Compensation Commission	One of many terms identifying the state public body which administers the workers' compensation laws, holds hearings on contested cases, promotes industrial safety, rehabilitation, etc. It is often located within the state labor department. The national organization is the International Association of Industrial Accident Boards and Commissions.

BIBLIOGRAPHY

Terms and definitions appearing in this GLOSSARY were drawn, in part, from the following publications and communications:

American Speech-Language-Hearing Association: Definitions, 1982-1988. (Excerpted from definitions provided by the American Speech-Language Hearing Association, 1801 Rockville Park, Rockville, MD, 20852)

Apter S, Mintz-Bitman S, Cooper S, et al: Brain Injury: A Family Guide. Philadelphia, PA, Magee Rehabilitation Hospital, 1986

Becker DP, Povlishock JT (eds): Central Nervous System Trauma Status Report. Bethesda National Institute of Neurological and Communication Disorders and Stroke, 1985

Bruckner EE and Randle APH: Return to work after severe head injuries. Rheumatology & Physical Medicine, 11:344-348, 1972

Berrol S: Personal communication, dated June 10, 1988

Cooper PR (ed): Head Injury. Baltimore, MD, Williams and Wilkins, 1982

Dresser AC, Meirowsky AM, Weiss GH, et al: Gainful employment following head injury. Archives of Neurology, 29:111-116, 1973

Gibbs J and Bell KE: Rehabilitation in head injury - A case study. Rehabilitation Nursing 12:137-138, 1987

Heaton RK, Chelune GJ and Lebman RAW: Using neuropsychological and personality tests to assess the likelihood of patient employment. Journal of Nervous and Mental Disorders, 166:408-416, 1978

Jennett B and Teasdale G: Management of Head Injuries. Philadelphia, PA, FA Davis, 1981

Kreutzer J, Lent B, Coulter S and McNeny R: A glossary of cognitive rehabilitation terminology. Cognitive Rehabilitation 4(3):10-13, 1986

Levin H and Grossman RG: Behavioral sequelae of closed head injury. Archives of Neurology, 35:720-727, 1978

Matkin RE, Insurance Rehabilitation. Austin, Texas, Pro-Ed Inc., 1985

Marshall LF, Sadler GR and Marshall SB: Head Injury. San Diego, CA, The Central Nervous System Injury Foundation, 1981, pp 16, 26-28 (Available from The Central Nervous System Injury Foundation, 4050 Front Street, San Diego, CA 92103)

McNeil MR: Current concepts in adult aphasia. International Rehabilitation Medicine 6:128-134, 1984

National Head Injury Foundation: Glossary. Undated, printed (Obtained from the National Head Injury Foundation, 333 Turnpike Road, Southborough MA 01772)

Newman OS, Heatch RK and Lehman RAW: Neuropsychological and MMPI correlates of patients' future employment characteristics. Perceptual and Motor Skills, 46:635-642, 1978

Rosenthal M (ed): Glossary of Neuropsychological Terms. National Head Injury Foundation, 333 Turnpike Rd., Southborough, MA, 1985

Santa Clara Valley Medical Center Head Injury Service: Coma Inservice Glossary. Undated, mimeographed, (Obtained from SCVMC Head Injury Service, Santa Clara Valley Medical Center, 751 South Bascom Avenue, San Jose, CA 95128)

Santa Clara Valley Medical Center Head Injury Service: Selected Terms. Undated, mimeographed, pp 18-24 (Obtained from SCVMC Head Injury Service, Santa Clara Valley Medical Center, 751 South Bascom Avenue, San Jose, CA 95128)

Sarno MT, Buonaguro A and Levita E: Characteristics of verbal impairment in closed head injured patients. Archives of Physical Medicine and Rehabilitation 67:400-405, 1986

Soderback I, Normell A: Intellectual function training in adults with acquired brain damage. Scandinavian Journal of Rehabilitation Medicine 18:139-146, 1986

Source Book of Health Insurance Data 1981-1982, 23rd edition. Health Insurance Association of America, Washington, DC, 1982

Texas Head Injury Foundation: Comprehensive Rehabilitation of the Head-Injured Person: A Family Education Manual. 1986 (Available from the Texas Head Injury Association, 8911 Capitol of Texas Hwy., North, Building 4, Suite 4140, Austin, TX 78759)

Treasure Coast Rehabilitation Hospital: Glossary. Vero Beach, Center for Coma Management at Treasure Coast (From a syllabus distributed at a conference on "Coma Management: A Rehabilitation Perspective" held in Vero Beach, FL, December 11, 1987)

TIRR BRAIN INJURY GLOSSARY

Vogenthaler DR: An overview of head injury: Its consequences and rehabilitation. Brain Injury 1:113-127, 1987

The editor is grateful to the many additional individuals who provided suggestions for revision of the first draft of this Glossary. Barry Willer, PhD, Rehab RT Center - TBI, SUNY Buffalo, shared copies of glossaries he had collected but which cannot be properly credited because the origins are unknown.